I0781849

DIARY OF A MARATHON

To my kids

*Because sometimes running a marathon
is more relaxing than parenting*

Love you both!

Introduction

When I was in high school, I once ran for an entire quarter of a mile without stopping.

They had to send me to the nurse's office.

I was always a walk-the-straights, run-the-curves kind of girl, except when I had the option to skip the running part. I absolutely never ran when my grade wasn't dependent on it.

Once I had escaped the tortuous requirements of high school Phys Ed, I tried taking up running exactly three more times. On occasion I would see a runner along the side of the road, that beautiful form dancing in forward motion, and think it looked like fun. So, once in college, I got up early and went out for a jog. I stepped out of the Quad into the cool morning air, nothing but taxi drivers and delivery vans on the street, and started to jog. I'm pretty sure I had passed almost two buildings before realizing this was a stupid idea, turning around, and walking home.

The following summer, my sometime-boyfriend was trying to get into shape to be a lifeguard at the beach. His routine included running, so I opted to join him. Having a crush makes you do silly things, like run-walk routines in too-tight shoes for nearly a mile through town until the tops of your feet hurt so badly you can hardly walk. At the time I was working at a three-story bed-and-breakfast and had to go up and down the stairs dozens of times each day - backwards, sitting down, because my feet hurt so badly. Beautiful forward-dancing creature I was not.

Years later, in graduate school, I decided to do the same thing. My soon-to-be husband had started taking an occasional run, and I thought I would join him. By then I didn't even own a sports bra, so I figured I would skip the underwires I did own and run free. By the end of our jog, I was lumping along with my arms held tightly across my chest, cursing the traffic, the narrowness of the shoulder we were running along, my ill-fitting shoes, the word "flop", my obviously twisted fiance, and the very pastime of running. I forgave my fiance, eventually, but that was the last time I would try anything as stupid as going out for a run.

Maybe running was good for some people; it clearly was not for me. Over a decade passed before I had any urge to try again. I got married, moved across the country, had two babies, and started a surreal life as a stay-at-home mom (something I swore I would NEVER do). My sister-in-law Cathy became a runner. Her weight had gotten high enough that, on accompanying me to one of my final OB visits prior to giving birth to my daughter, she was disturbed to realize she weighed more than I did at 9+ months pregnant. She turned her life completely around and started running the track at the high school where she taught. She started out run-walking. Then she ran more. And more. She started signing up for races (an easy thing to do where we live in Tucson, Arizona). She completed a half marathon. Then another. It wasn't long before she set her sights on a full. I told her people have to be nuts to attempt a full marathon; this was something I swore I would NEVER do (I need to learn to stop saying that.). But she did it! She lost eighty pounds of weight, gained twice that weight in confidence, and ran the San Francisco Marathon. She went on to run at least one marathon every year. She was truly inspirational. One would think she would be what inspired me, but my mind doesn't work that easily. Seeing the amazing things she did never incited in me a desire to be amazing too.

Nope. What inspired me was Boston. THAT Boston. The BAD Boston. April 2013. Watching the news on television as it broke, seeing the smoke, the blood, the faces that were either terrified or completely blank as they stood shaking near the finish line, I saw the gantry. My very first clear thought was, "So that's a marathon finish line. I want to do that some day."

Clearly I should have gone directly to a shrink's office, but instead I went to the YMCA. We already had a family membership there, and I was already walking on the treadmill multiple times a week. For once, though, I set the speed a little higher. I put it all the way up to 5.0. That's a 12-minute mile. I knew I'd managed faster than that for that first quarter mile way back in high school (I had managed to finish run-walking a 10'22" before crashing that day), so I decided to keep it up for a quarter of a mile. I was wearing men's hiking shoes, yoga pants, a cotton shirt, and a regular bra, but I did it. After that, I walked until the treadmill read 3.1 miles. Maybe I can do a 5k one day?

I moved slowly - both as far as running pace and as far as incrementally increasing the amount of running I did. By May of 2013, I was able to run-walk a treadmill 5k in 40 minutes, 21 seconds. My husband found out I had started running and nearly fainted. By the end of the month, I got fitted for actual running shoes and ran outside for the first time. On June 19, I did 5k on the treadmill with no walking breaks. I sent a note to my sister-in-law: I was ready to do a real 5k race with her.

She and I were planning a trip to New Jersey that summer, so she signed us up for a 5k there. At the last minute, the race was canceled. "Not to worry," she exclaimed, "I found a 5-miler that's even closer!"

I thought she was insane to believe I could ever manage five miles when I was still struggling to finish three. And yet there I found myself, standing at the start line of a tiny race in Avalon, New Jersey. It was a complete foreign country for me. I didn't even know where to pin my bib. To add to the surrealness, a bank of fog had overtaken the town so that we could hardly see two or three houses ahead. I would never have done it without her; I would have driven home and hid under my bed. I started out too fast, which is a popular error, I suppose. I couldn't manage to run the full five miles. I walked some. She stayed with me. I ran some, and she stayed with me. I walked some more. The last leg took us up onto the slippery dew-coated boardwalk. By now there was just one person behind us. I know this because, as we got up onto the boardwalk, a volunteer asked if we were "it". Cathy's answer of "one guy behind us" was met with an eyeroll and a sigh that this volunteer's duty was not quite finished. And then, next thing I knew, the finish line was in sight. My goal was to finish in less than an hour; the clock read 59:30. With a burst of energy, I sprinted in for that dramatic finish. Cathy could easily have left me in the dust (well, sand), but she let me go first. Waiting to cheer us at the finish were my parents, grandmother, and kids; I had as many cheerleaders as there were miles in this little race! I never even saw what my official time was (the race was so small it was gun-timed only), nor did I honestly care.

So, I couldn't actually RUN for the entirety of my first race, and it was only five miles. I felt no urge to let that stop me. I just kept working. After a while, I COULD run for 5 miles nonstop. Then six. Seven. I made a deal with myself.

If I could run eight miles, I could surely do a half marathon.
And I did.

So here I was, having only raced once before and
having been unable to actually run that entirely, watching as
my fingers signed up for the Tucson Half Marathon in
December. I carefully wrote out a training plan. I vowed not
to tell my husband until the last possible moment (or until
Cathy accidentally mentioned it over dinner one evening) so
he wouldn't point out the audacity of this idea. Race
morning came, and with Cathy by my side, I boarded a
school bus for the first time in 16 years. It drove us an
astronomically long distance through the dark desert to the
start line, where it proceeded to snow. Hell freezing over,
snow in the desert, me running a half marathon - all about
the same likelihood. But I did! I walked a bit toward the end,
but I finished with a respectable time of 2:28:53 and received
my first and most treasured finisher's medal. I looked over
at Cathy and realized that she was most assuredly some
sort of alien creature for ever having done this distance
TWICE in a ROW. I would never do that. (Did I mention I
should never say that?)

I was soon introduced to the many races put on
around Tucson. I could do a race every weekend if I wanted.
I opted to stick to some of the races put on by the Southern
Arizona Roadrunners. I even did a 10k all by myself - my
first race without Cathy - and started to feel more confident.

I knew I would never win, but pushing through to the finish line and seeing the race bibs collect on my counter was getting me hooked.

I went back to New Jersey for the summer and ran in my hometown race for the first time. The town of Cape May Point puts on a 2-mile and 5-mile race in June. Up until now, the extent of my participation involved selling baked goods to benefit my church at the staging area and ogling the group of Coast Guards who would always come to do the 2-mile in gorgeous uniform. Standing at the start line of the 5-mile, I felt like two people. Was I the hometown girl who never ran? Or the exotic half-marathoner from the desert southwest?

It turned out I was the one who had just driven solo across the entire country in a small car full of kids and dogs; I fought hard to maintain my mediocre 11-something pace. But doing that race, crossing THAT finish line, I really felt for the first time, I felt like a Runner.

The following November, back in Tucson, I did another local half marathon, the Veteran's Day Half Marathon put on by another local group called Everyone Runs. It was a bit of a roller coaster of a course, but I ran the entire time - my first time ever - and finished in 2:30:50. I found it ironic that I had not walked at all and yet still finished a bit slower than my previous race, but I blamed the hills.

A few weeks later, I was back at the Tucson Half Marathon. A year had passed before this First Big Race of mine. I was excited to see how different it might feel. Even though I had only done it once before, the course felt familiar. I knew there was one hill, and I was ready for it. I had vowed the previous year that I would be The Coolest Runner and run up the hill, and I did - only to be absolutely out of energy at the top and find myself having to walk for a mile or so. With age comes wisdom. I planned to walk the hill, and that was all I walked - I ran the entire rest of the race. My final time was 2:29:29. I was happy to know my times were consistent, but the fact that they were so consistent whether I ran or walked was a bit mystifying. Although my time was essentially the same, though, my body felt different. Whereas the previous year I felt like an overdone slice of toast, this year I felt fine. I had energy to spare. I could have - gasp - kept going.

And so there I found myself the very next day, reading the race director's "sign up now for next year and save money!" email, moving my mouse pointer over, and clicking on Race: FULL.

I was in.

Since I had signed up for a race that was a full year away, I was able to attempt to forget such a nonsensical move for a while. I ran more 10k's, more 5k's, and even another lovely half with another running friend.

As I had for my half marathon, I had carefully perused the Internet in search for the training plan that had the least terms I would need to Google. (Fartlek? Interval? Stride?

Tempo? What?) I found one, dutifully printed it out, and taped it to the refrigerator. A few oddly timed and oddly distanced runs later, it was time to start.

The First Few Miles

July 12

Technically my first day of training. It's a day I can handle, because it's a rest day. I spend the day just chasing around my kids, and the four others we have staying at my house for the weekend. Six kids under 6. If I can handle this, I can handle a marathon.

July 13

Oh, I have to run to train for a marathon? Still, it's an easy day. Only five miles. I've done five miles too many times before to count. This is different than my usual five miles, however. I'm starting my training in New Jersey, which has the benefit of being only double-digit degrees at any time of day, clouds that block the sun that normally combusts any runners out past 6:30am like a bully frying ants. The drawback is that there is humidity. My first training run is through soup, and within a quarter mile I am a soggy noodle floating through it. I don't start running until just after 8am. This is running on vacation.

I bring along the dog. I don't want to bring along the dog, because while she likes running and I like running, she and I do not like running together. Having assumed we had long since agreed on this point, I left her home last week while I went for a quick run and returned to hear that she had sat with her nose fogging up the door crying the entire time I was gone. I am left with the choice of bringing the dog or a load of guilt. I opt for dog. She is relatively polite for me this time, pooping within a few yards of the sole trash can on my route, and only trying to flip me over once when she confused my "let's cross the street and turn back for home" command with "HOLYCRAP THERE'S A RABBIT IN THAT FIELD LET'S CHASE IT!"

The strange thing with running where I grew up is that I see people I know, and it's funny how they all seem to float by while I'm running. I see Bill. Hi, Bill. I see Ralph. Hi, Ralph. I see a Green Heron. I don't technically know the Green Heron, but this being Cape May, one of THE birding destinations, it's fun to see something that would never have popped up on my dry-wash runs in Tucson. Hi, Green Heron.

My pace today is 10:26. This is too fast for me. I am out of breath, and this was supposed to be an easy run. I even managed a 10-minute mile. I'd pat myself on the back, but if I work this hard on my easy runs, I'll die on my hard ones.

July 14

    Cross-training day. I'm sure they mean something like cycling, swimming, or elliptical, but I opt for yoga. I've gone from a five-day-a-week rubber-band-lady yoga junkie to a once-in-a while used-to-be-able-to-reach-that girl. Yoga has helped me through training injuries before, and figuring that training for twice the distance will lead to twice the injuries (how's that for some newbie running math?), I will use my cross-training day to nip that in the bud. Not to mention I seriously hate cycling, swimming, and elliptical. I park my mat on my "yoga loft" (an area of the house that every person has named for their own use) and get into the most pathetic pigeon I've done in a year. I rise, begin to change position, and the dog comes and plops down directly behind me on the mat. Yeesh, dog.

July 15

    Only four miles. If I could handle bringing the dog for five, why not four? So along she comes. We get a tenth of a mile from my house and she poops. I'm too grumpy to turn around and bring it back to my house, so we run on toward that sole public trash can. I get around the corner from there and see Charlotte. Hi, Charlotte. We have a five-minute chat. I might just love running at home. Having gotten an earlier start, there are a dozen other runners out and about. Most of them are probably people on vacation. These are True Runners. You must be a True Runner if you run on vacation. I don't get a chance to talk to any of them since they pass me too quickly, but it makes me feel less out-of-place. Cape May has plenty of birdwatching events, but the running events are few and far between.

We get to the two-mile turn-around. I pause to let traffic get past. The dog poops again. I am as far from the trash can as I can be, and there's that squishy pile mocking me. I dutifully clean it up, then run along with the dog leash in one hand (I haven't figured out how to swing my arms with the leash) and a bag of poo in the other. The humidity of the morning is causing a thick coat of slime to form between my hand and the bag. I pass a tempting number of residential trash cans. Still, I grasp my slimy bag with an ethical clench. We eventually make it to the public trash can. I doubt the sight of the finish line will be as delightful as the sight of the trash can. The rest of the way around the lake, and we're home. I wash my hands. A lot.

My pace is 10:37. I am happy with that.

July 16

Six miles to do today. There's no way I could bring the dog and maintain some shred of sanity, so she stays home with the promise that my mom will give her nibbles of bacon if she starts to cry. It only takes one nibble to make today a good day for the dog.

I haven't run six miles since the beginning of May, or, as my legs see it, "never". Still, there is the excitement of covering new territory. In my previous runs, I had gone around the west side of the lake that's near my house, a long, vaguely comma-shaped lake called Lake Lily; that adds an extra three-quarters of a mile. Today, I head up the east side for a short time before I make my easterly turn onto Seagrove Avenue. The town was once called Seagrove, and now we have this lovely avenue in memorium to that. Seagrove Ave has the added benefit of the tiniest percentage of the traffic I'd find on my only other possible route, Sunset Boulevard. Sunset is a haphazard mass of Real Runners on their vacation runs, cars that remember when the speed limit was 50, cars that are too excited by the view to speed all the way up to the new limit of 35, tourists on rented bicycles, and 10-foot-wide lawn service vehicles parked on the 2-foot-wide shoulder. Sleepy Seagrove does just fine by me.

My noncommittal legs suddenly get a burst of interest in what I am telling them to do when I realize I will actually reach the canal. I have never run as far as the canal before, so this feels like a major feat. It's a perfect 5k from my front door to the closest view of the canal, at the end of a delightfully forested dead end road.

It takes my legs about five miles to warm up (marathons were made for folk like me), so on the return I get a sudden burst of energy and start to feel like I actually am a runner. The bacon-sated dog forgives me as I walk in the door. 10:44 average pace. Not too shabby.

July 17

A day of rest! I do enjoy these.

The First Long Runs

July 18

My first official long-run day. I still snicker at the official training plan I have taped to the fridge - LSD. That's Long Slow Distance. Today's LSD run is just another six miles, so I head back out to the canal and back. It's easier heading out this time since I know I'll be rewarded at my turn-around point. My legs are tired, but I manage a 10:49 pace. As a bonus, I run into another friend at the foot of the lake on my return, so I get to chat with him for a bit. After that few minutes rest, I run the last block to my house. My feet feel like they have turned into a pair of elephants. Remind me never to stop for this long on a run again.

In the evening, my best childhood friend arrives for the week to visit her family. They stop by our house. I tell her I'm training for a marathon. Knowing how much I've always hated running, she looks at me as if I've grown two heads. She may be right.

July 19

Rest day after my long run.

July 20

Today was scheduled to be a five-mile run. I think it's more of a five-mile swim. 91% humidity, and already 80-degrees when I hit the pavement, I feel like I'm jogging through thick soup. I eke out an 11:13 average pace and come back dripping as if I'd just run the full marathon in 2:30.

July 21

Cross-training day. My plan was to do yoga, but I spend the day holding onto the dog as she quivers in terror at the thunderstorms that come through to cut that humidity.

July 22

An easy four miles. I decide to take the dog again; I know I can handle her for four miles. We dash through the no-longer-humid air, rounding the west side of the lake again (there's that lovely poop disposal bin on the far side), up Seagrove, across Sunset and into West Cape May. It is here that we pick up the extra dog. A big fluffy husky comes out of a yard, and there is much butt-sniffing. My normally excruciatingly submissive dog (she has flipped to show her belly to 4-week-old puppies) seems happy to have made a friend. I see no humans that may belong to this dog, so I say, "Go home!" and start up running again. Extra Dog comes with. She runs with us for a while, looking so happy at this fact that I haven't the heart to tell her not to. Eventually she gives us a thank-you wag and runs up into another yard.

As we near our turn-around point, I frighten another woman out running with her dog. I don't mean to. We turned onto the road she was running on, just a few feet behind her and on the other side of the road. She doesn't have a clue we're there, as she has her headphones on. I tell my dog that it's time for us to turn around. Her dog hears and turns to come with us; it is then that she realizes we're there. She yells angrily at her dog. I can only imagine what she's thinking, seeing us coming up behind her and then turning back suddenly as soon as we see that she's aware of us.

The dog drags me through the streets. She's so used to my husband's pace that she surely doesn't count this as a "run". Between the free pull and the delightfully lower humidity, we do a 10:23 pace. I even manage a mile at 10:01. I rock! (In my own slow-runner way…)

July 23

Time to try this six miler again. I get a later start since my kids have slept in (something they don't do on days when I don't have a run, of course). It is sunny, but not actually hot. The desert runner in me is overreacting to the sun, so I have to keep reminding myself that "sunny" does not equal "hot". The first week of training has paid off, and my legs feel quite happy to just roll along the road. I get up to the canal, turn back, and notice a large feather. REALLY large feather. It's at least eight inches long. I pick it up and stick it in my pony tail, sticking up so I look like some sort of blond-haired, blue-eyed Indian. For the remaining three miles, every runner and cyclist who passes me giggles.

In Tucson I usually run with earbuds, but that has seemed the less-than-optimal choice here. For one, I own cheap earbuds (I do love the dollar bins at Target), so with the added humidity, they ooze their way continuously out of my ears. I also run on the roads here, as opposed to on a bike path in Tucson, so I have to be able to hear if a car is coming. In lieu of earbuds, I have just had my music playing in my belt. I figure I spent so little time within hearing range of any other humans, they could probably handle a few seconds of my odd mix of sea chanties and Meat Loaf. This has worked for the past two weeks.

Except today. It just so happened today that a nice old man was out walking his cocker spaniel (a breed of dog that seemed to make this man both nicer and older). He was heading toward me, so I prepared my winning, feather-hatted smile… just as that One Song on my playlist popped up. Bloodhound Gang began to sing.

"The roof. The roof. The roof is on fire"

Uh-oh. I start to reach for the zipper of my belt pack.

The old man draws nearer.

"The roof. The roof. The roof is on fire."

Zipper. Can't get the zipper open. Why can't I get the zipper open? Why??

"The roof. The roof. The roof is on fire."

Got the zipper to open at last. I grab for my phone only to realize I have opened it all of a half an inch, and no iPhone would ever squeeze out of that space. Kindly old man smiles the churchiest smile at me. I have now pulled my shirt halfway up my body, swung my belt about as high as my neck in my attempt to pull the offending phone out, and am probably making a face befitting a mouse about to give birth to a walrus. Is it just me, or did I just crank the volume up as high as it will go?

"We don't need no water, let the mother-fu--"
"GOOD MORNING, SIR!" I yell so loudly I almost knock him over. A moment later I finally have figured out once again how zippers work, pull the phone out, and give it a look of delightfully dramatic offense, and advance to the next song.

That went smoothly.

Pace: 10:55. Heart rate: 2000.

July 24

A day to rest up before my long run on Saturday. Or, a day to reconfigure my playlist. Either way…

The Angriest Son

July 25

Eight miles today. For once I set an alarm to get up early, rather than wait for my kids to wake up and be content before I go. I'm on the road by 6:15. It's wonderfully lonely on the roads, and a light mist is rising from the fields as I pass them. The birds are singing loudly. Why have I not gotten up this early before?

Instead of heading straight to the canal, I turn left before that last dead-end section of road and head toward Higbee's Beach. Higbee's Beach is known for two things: bird-watchers and nudity. The beach was the only nude beach for years, legally and otherwise, but it also has a perfect habitat for the slew of birds that filter through Cape May on their fall migration. On a typical late-summer day, one would find a beach full of naked folks surrounded by a forest full of folks with binoculars. These days, it's rare to find the full moon on the beach, but the bird watchers are still going strong. I reach the parking area for the birders and turn onto a little dirt road that leads to the dike. The dike is a huge pile of sand covered in phragmities, next to which is a wooden platform. On that platform, for the entirety of the fall migration season, there will be a guy whose entire job is to count the number of each species that flies over in the dawn's early light. These are serious birders. This morning there is just one man on the platform. I must make my footfalls as quiet as possible. In all those decades, the birders were never moved to turn their binoculars toward the nudists, but they would surely beat me with them should I accidentally scare off something rare.

On the way back, I almost get hit by a car. It's the paper delivery man. He is known for driving very old cars. He has at least two of them, and he rotates them as a good runner rotates shoes. Normally I can smell his cars before I see them, and the scent lingers longer than the time it takes to read the Sunday paper. This time I can hear him. There's a blind turn from West Avenue onto Stevens Street in West Cape May. There's a stop sign on West, but at that time of morning I know there is an expectation that no cars will be in the way should a driver decide to blow the stop. This morning I can hear the clunk of his car as he comes up West, so I move way over onto the grass to give him lots of room. He flies around the corner, two wheels on the tiny shoulder, and by the time he notices me it would have been way too late to stop. I was prepared for this, so I smile and wave. He is too busy panicking that he was about to hit me to realize that he didn't, and that I'm smiling at him. He drives past with adrenalin-widened eyes.

I have found a pace that feels like cruising gear. I float happily over the roads on my return trip. I get home before my son even wakes up, which is a very good thing. At three years old, he is not impressed by my running. At all. He does wake up a few minutes after I get home and instantly screams at me to take my shirt off (he knows a running shirt when he sees one). I do. (Hey, I'm wearing a running bra, it's cool!) When I sit next to him and tell him I've already gone for the run, he screams at me that I'm all sweaty and need to take a shower. I do. All is forgiven.

11:11 pace. Yes, I'm slow. It's okay.

July 26

Rest day. No soreness from my "long" run yesterday, so that's nice.

July 27

Five miles. There was a tiny bit of rain in the morning, and we had some errands to run "in town" (Cape May proper). When it's summer and it rains, the tourists generally get in their cars and drive around in slow, pointless circles, occasionally stopping to go into stores to wander around in slow, pointless circles. We opt to go run our errands first, before everyone else wakes up enough to realize it's a rainy day. We get back from our errands at 10:00, and I dress to go for a run. At 10:15. In July. It's lovely to not be in Tucson.

Since there are still some thunderstorms in the area, I stick to Cape May Point. It's a very small town, so I have to run around the entire town - twice - to make five miles. I see at least a dozen other runners, some of them multiple times. Here we are, running around in slow, pointless circles.

10:58 per mile. Hey, at least it's under 11.

July 28

Yoga day! And I actually DO yoga today. It feels awesome.

July 29

Five miles again. I take the dog. We do the Cape May Point loop again. It's pretty hot and humid, so the dog and I are both slow with our tongues hanging out. The dog is having a lot of fun looking around. So much so that she runs face-first into a no-parking sign. On the second loop, we pass a family of Mute Swans. The dog is a bird dog. The Mute Swans are birds. I am no longer running with a dog; I am now holding a leash attached to a 30-pound vibrating rock. I manage to get her to stop pointing the swans. A few yards down the road, we catch up to my friend Anita. I stop to chat. The dog is no longer running with a human; she is now at the end of a leash attached to a 140-pound chatty human. Smarter than me, she just takes the opportunity to stretch out.

We finish up the run with an average 10:43 pace. I'm so sweaty, my fingers are pruny before I even get in the shower.

July 30

Six mile day. Back to the Canal. The run out is calm, but on the way back I hear the fire siren in West Cape May. A few minutes later, I hear the fire siren in Cape May Point. Being far away and without a way to get home faster, I'm sure it's my house that's on fire, especially when I see the fire truck head toward Cape May Point. My pace quickens to a 10:30 mile as I chase the fire truck. It slows to 11:09 when I see the Cape May Point fire truck heading back from the call, well north of my house. My favorite kind of drama is the kind that isn't actually dramatic.

10:50 per mile.

July 31

Rest day. I spend the morning making pies, cupcakes, and muffins I have no plan of eating. They are to be donated to our church bazaar, which is tomorrow. Somehow the training has caught up with me, though, so several of the cupcakes end up not making it to the church.

The Earliest Mornings

August 1

Bazaar Day. This is the longest day of the year for my family. It is also the day my training plan has a 9-mile run scheduled. So far I have done every run exactly as scheduled, so I decide to stick to the plan. My alarm goes off at still-dark o'clock. I sneak past my son, who is sleeping on the floor next to the bed (we also have a houseguest for the weekend, who is sleeping in my son's room, hence the floor campout). I get out the door without waking him up, so I already feel like I have won. Go, me.

I sneak out the back door into the dark morning. There's a full moon, so it's not too dark. I can almost see the sky start to lighten in the east. It's a beautiful time to run. Also dangerous. My town is a town full of skunks. It's not long before I see a shadowy form start to cross the road in front of me. It's too dark to tell what it is. It is followed by another. And another. After the fourth I am now close enough to see that they are just raccoons. After the sixth, I am starting to be nervous that I will soon be eaten by the raccoon posse. Thankfully the lead raccoon sees me, gives a chirp to her teens, and they all turn back and scurry into the bushes from whence they had come. Crisis averted.

The birds at this time of morning are deafening. There are warblers that land in the center of the street and sing. Dark forms in a dark street singing their light song.

The sun finally starts thinking about rising as I pass Rea's Farm in West Cape May. A chorus of roosters in the distance make sure I notice this.

I make a few different turns so that I end up running along the Canal for a bit. The fresh salt air makes me feel like I could go on forever. As I go along New England Road toward Higbee's, the paper delivery man drives by. Lots of distance between us this time. I smile and wave. He does not. I don't mind.

By the time I turn back, other folks are starting to wake up. I run past the household of the folks who are in charge of running the Bazaar this morning. They are busily loading up their cars with last-minute supplies. I shout out a hearty "Good morning! I'll be there in three miles!" Marty asks if I want a ride. It's hard to say no, but I do.

A giant orange sun is rising into the trees as I get back home. A quick shower, and it's off to work. Everyone else is just getting themselves awake enough to start the day, and I've already run nine miles. I like this feeling.

10:51 pace. That's pretty awesome.

August 2

Rest day. My left leg is a bit sore, but I'm too busy with church and houseguests and kids to really pay it any mind.

August 3

Things are ramping up; I have a six mile run on my training calendar for today. I like the six mile runs, though. The Canal doesn't seem as far away as it used to.

My husband is here now. I was excited to have him here so that I could get up early to avoid the sun, go for my run, and not make my mom listen for my son. Instead, my husband announces that he wants to get up and run too. He plans on going 8 miles. He plans on getting up at 6. We opt to both get up at 6am. I joke that I'll still be doing my six miles while he does his eight miles. He takes the dog with him, however; he actually likes running with the dog. The dog poops so early into his run that he doubles back to drop the baggie into our trash can. I am almost half a mile into my run by the time he catches up. Amazingly, I finish my run before him. That means I get to shower first, too. Woohoo!

10:48 pace.

August 4

Yoga day. I love yoga. Wish I'd gotten around to doing it today.

August 5

Six miles. My husband is running this morning too. I let him get up first and don't get out of bed until he is ready to leave. He and the dog are gone by the time I'm dressed and ready to head out.

I'm out at sunrise. There are some clouds leftover from last night's thunderstorms, which make for a beautiful sunrise. On Seagrove I pass the same dark warblers that had been singing from the middle of the street, and they are just as dark at dawn as they had been in the earlier morning. So, not warblers at all. Indigo Buntings? Or Blue Grosbeaks. I always get them mixed up.

The farm stand on Bayshore Road opened a few days ago. I can smell their peaches as I run by. They smell fantastic.

The paper delivery man drives past. I wave at him. He waves back to me this time. Things are looking up.

As I get to the Canal, I can hear footsteps behind me. Then a jackass comes up and asks me to hold his dog while he goes to pee in the woods. Wait, that's my dog. And my jackass! I make sure to give the dog back to him before he runs off. He is so fast, I lose sight of him before I even get to the intersection with New England Road.

Back on Stevens Street, I hear the paper delivery man's car coming around the blind corner again. I get onto the grass quickly, and he shoots around the corner again. I wave again. He is gone to quickly for me to see his reaction this time.

When I get to the foot of the lake, I see the husband and dog walking up ahead. They do not see me. Husband makes for the back door. I rush my way into the front door so I can take up a very nonchalant seat in the living room. "Gee, you're slow," I say as he comes in. The look of shock and confusion is worth every drip of sweat I'm getting on this chair.

My son is still asleep. In lieu of a shower, I take a quick rinse and change into horseback riding clothes. When he wakes up and sees me in breeches, he is excited. He knows he'll get to go riding too. Riding is much more fun than running. I hope my legs aren't too tired to keep me on the horse.

10:29 pace. I actually went 6.2 miles. If I hadn't walked the last half a block, that would have been my fastest 10k.

August 6

Five long, horse-sore miles. I don't understand how my inner thigh muscles have apparently never done any work while running, judging by how flaccid they were yesterday, but now that they are sore from riding they seem to be the only muscles required.

I lump my way around Cape May Point. 10:37 pace. When I get home to take a shower, I can hardly get up the stairs.

August 7

Day off. Phew.

August 8

Another day for a long run. Today it's 10 miles. I get up before dawn, but I'm actually the third person to leave for a workout; my husband and father have already left for a long bike ride by the time I get out the door. One would think we were a family of health nuts. We are not. At all.

I am completely not in the mood to run. It's a small miracle that I get out the door. It takes me a while to get my brain into the idea. The rising sun catches some fantastic clouds, painting just the bottom curves of each one a lovely rosey pink. My mood brightens with the day. My legs are not as sore, and by the time I hit mile 3 ("almost" half-way), this all seems doable.

I seem to have paced myself just right; I average 10:54 but my last mile is the fastest, at 10:22. Maybe it was the sinister number of vultures I passed on my return trip, or the welcoming thought of the company at my house. This weekend it's my aunt and my paternal grandmother. I get to gorge on cucumbers from their garden when I get back. Why is it that a storebought cucumber tastes nothing like the ones fresh from the garden? They should give these out at race water stations.

August 9

Time to rest after my long miles yesterday. And eat more cucumbers.

August 10

This is a multi-use run. Five miles of marathon training, yes, but also a pre-burn of calories for tonight. This afternoon we're taking the ferry down to Delaware for a pilgrimage to the Dogfish Head Brewpub, where I will eat all the foods. So, also five miles to earn all the foods. I run the double loop around town. It's relatively hot today, so I'm slow. 11:06 average pace.

August 11

Cross-training day. I get to sleep in after my fantastic evening of gluttony, then do yoga in the afternoon. My favorite style is Yin yoga. It's all about holding positions for long periods of time and with little muscle effort, so the fascia surrounding your muscles can stretch. It's a wonderful thing for runners to do to avoid chronic compartment syndrome. It's also nice on days when I hardly feel like being awake. I get into a good position and hold it. I wake up about 20 minutes later with the longest, loosest fascia ever.

I do end up going for a "run" in the evening. A big storm is rolling in, so I head up to the lake to watch some amazing clouds come blowing in. I watch, and watch, and watch. Then the storm actually arrives. There is lightning striking everywhere and giant balls of rain smashing down.

Somehow I had forgotten that part of a good storm. I stand dazed for a moment, then run like a maniac back to my house.

August 12

To the Canal and back; six miles. The storm cut through the humidity, so this run feels much better than the last few. I rock a 10:45 pace.

August 13

Just five miles today. I had planned to run the whole time around my friend Bob's house. He hates runners and says they flaunt their runs right at him. He and my husband are out fishing, though, so I just stick to my traditional double loop. 10:46 pace.

August 14

I do love these rest days.

August 15

A "short" long run today - eight miles. I'm tired, so I decide to not set an alarm. I'll just sleep in and go for my run whenever I wake up. Which I do, promptly at 5:45. D'oh!

A nice mouthful of peanut butter, and I'm on my way. The air is very cool this morning. It's quiet on the streets, except for the twittering of birds coming through. Mid-August is the start of the fall migration here, so there are birders all around chasing those birds. The lot at the Beanery is full. It used to be, of all things, a beanery (lima beans, to be specific), but now it's overgrown and intensely popular with fall birders. The lot down at Higbee's is half full, as well. Tomorrow is the first official day of counting bird species from the Dike. Today must be the soft opening.

West Cape May smells like peas today. There are still a lot of farms tucked back here, although several of them have turned into housing developments. I want to find the peas and eat them.

The paper delivery man drives past me twice. He doesn't hit me either time. He waves. He's driving his 30-year-old white car today. I can smell it for several minutes each time he passes me. I love the smell of old cars.

11:01 pace. Lame, perhaps, but my last mile was also my fastest. At least I'm doing that part right.

August 16

Rest!

August 17

Six miles, to the Canal and back. Partway there, another runner comes from the opposite direction at an intersection and turns to run in the same direction as me. I assume I already look like something the cat threw up, but this other runner asks me if this is the road to Higbee Beach. I am honored that I have it together enough for other runners to trust me with directions. I tell her it's up the road we've just turned onto, then the first left, which is about a mile and a half away. She says thank you, and I dutifully slow down for a moment so she can run ahead of me. I am further shocked when I realize that she has the same pace as I do. This is the first time I've come across another runner out here who is not infinitely faster than me. Even more amazing, when we hit a few slight inclines (West Cape May has a low point of 0' above Sea Level to a high of oh, say, about 3' above Sea Level. Truly mountainous. But really, there are a few inclines!), I start to catch up with her. She slows down on the inclines more than I do! I am an Amazing Runner! After the one "large" hill, I realize that there is now a big housing development where one of the beautiful farm fields used to be, so it is now actually the second left my fellow runner must take. By now, in my blaze of awesomeness, I am close enough to her that I apologize for my old-timey-ness and tell her it's the second left. She says it looks familiar now. I ask her where she started from, and she names a spot at the far side of the next town over. She explains she decided to go out for a 2.5-hour run and had it timed just about right to go down to Higbee's and then back to her house to complete that run. So, she's basically at the last third of a half marathon, and I haven't quite hit three miles yet today. Bubble of awesomeness popped.

10:50 pace. In the afternoon, I drive my husband up to the airport so he can fly back to Tucson. Just a few more weeks here, and we'll have to go back too. Sigh.

August 18

Yoga day. By "yoga", I mean going up to get my oil changed and finding out that my brake line is busted. I wish my legs were as speedy as my car apparently is.

What Tempo Run?

August 19

    I wake up in the morning, ready to run my five miles today. It's my first tempo run in this training plan, so I want to be well-rested and fueled for it. My son sleeps in, but I figure I'd let him sleep and go for my run after he is settled. It's hot by the time he wakes up. It's hotter still by the time he's settled. I tell him I'm going for a run. He grumps a bit. I go up to get dressed. He busts the door down screaming before I even start. If only my husband were here, I could leave my little bundle of anger with him. I'm not willing to saddle my mom with that, though, so I change into civvies instead and stay home. I'll run in the afternoon when he feels better. He half-fusses for most of the morning and finally zonks on the couch around 1:45. It is now 85 degrees outside, with a heat index of 98. Now is my chance. I head out for my five miles. It does not feel good. There's no way I'm making this a tempo run. I take the dog, and she can't even keep up with my slow butt. I bring her back to the house after the first loop, then head out for the second half of my punishment. "Tempo run" is turning into "pathetic run-walk". As I pass St. Mary's, the Sisters of St. Joseph retreat, a nun hollers at me for running in this heat. You know it's bad if you're being yelled at by a nun. I drag myself home only to realize I'd miscalculated the part where I dropped the dog off and ended up running an extra quarter mile. Because I really needed to do that in this heat.

11:22 pace. There is not enough cold water in this world.

August 20

No matter what happens, I am NOT waiting until the heat of the afternoon to run today. Luckily my darling son is less fussy, so I get out at 9:30. Still later and hotter than I want, but at least it's not as bad as yesterday.

11:08 pace.

August 21

Rest day. It stormed from midnight to 4:00am, and the dog freaked out the whole time, so I'm extra glad I don't have to run today. And extra tired. But the storm cut that humidity, so life is good. Ready for a long one tomorrow. I make sure to drink lots of water so I'm ready for tomorrow.

August 22

Twelve miles. I set my alarm. Instead of rushing out the door, though, I relax with a cup of coffee, eat an R-Bar that my husband adamantly claimed as his own until he forgot to eat it or bring it back with him (ooh, double chocolate!), sip some water, then it's on the road right around sunrise. It's still early enough to see lots of wildlife. I pass a couple of raccoons crossing Seagrove Avenue in exactly the same spot I'd seen the family of raccoons crossing a few weeks ago. This time it's a little lighter, at least, so I don't have to slow down and wonder about shadowy forms being skunks.

Across Sunset Boulevard and into West Cape May. There is a large turkey in someone's yard. He is huge, with his chest puffed out, looking right at me. I remember my grandfather's attack turkey (to get to the front door you had to beat it away with a broom), so I quicken my pace a bit. This one does not attack.

I come across a little American Redstart, dead at the foot of someone's driveway. It's so tiny. You'd never guess how small they are as they flit around, but now that I'm up close to it, I'm amazed by how small it is. I stop and move it into some grass so the folks in the house don't have to come out to find such a tiny, sad sight.

My friend Mike is working in his garage as I pass their house. I say "good morning" in a voice that is much too cheerful for this early in the morning. He thinks I'm nuts. He's right.

Two guinea hens are in a field on one side of the street. A wishful cat is staring dreamily at them from the other side.

I reach the canal, but today I run toward the ocean instead of the bay. Today I am going over the bridge. The big, tall, getting taller and taller as I move toward it, bridge over the canal. It seems insurmountable. Then I surmount it. It's nowhere near as big as I had thought. I'm not quite five miles into the run when I hit the top, but it feels like I'm done. Funny how we build things up in our minds. I truck on down the other side, then run along the canal on the other side. The road eventually turns away from the canal and right to a McDonald's. I never thought hash browns could smell so delicious. Thank goodness I'm not carrying any cash. My six outbound miles take me nearly to the turnoff for the Ferry terminal. The road here is marked for the bike and/or run portions of the "Escape the Cape" triathlon, where competitors board the Ferry, ride it to the middle of the bay, then jump off and swim to shore for their first leg of the tri. It doesn't get any cooler than that! I slurp down a goo (Ooh, caramel macchiato! With hints of toasted marshmallow! Exquisite.), turn around, and remind myself slightly too late not to lick the sticky off my dead-bird-touching fingers. Eew.

I have been hydrating well, so I stop at a well-placed port-a-potty near a playground. While I'm in there, a car pulls up and someone gets out. There had been no other cars in the lot, so I'm sure the person has no clue that there's someone in the port-a-potty. I'm almost afraid to get out in case I scare him. I give him a minute to move farther away, then pop out and continue on my run.

Back up the bridge, a quick Rocky-esque dance at the top, then down through West Cape May. About two miles from home, my dad passes me. He's been out for a bike ride. It's funny that I've only passed four people on this whole run, and I've known half of them.

Across Sunset and into Cape May Point. I feel great. My pace is 10:57. Awesome!

August 23

Rest. And eat all the foods.

August 24

Six miles. I get a bit of a late start, but it's not too hot today. There are still puddles in some of the fields in West Cape May from the rain last week, and a number of Spotted Sandpipers are hanging out in one of the muddier puddles.

The water on the Canal is glassy. A fishing boat comes by, forming smooth waves in its wake. Next week is my last week here; after that I'll be lucky to have some brown, litter-filled water rushing down a wash right after a storm. No more perfectly glassy surfaces, no more fishing boats. I admit to tearing up a bit as I turn and head back home.

10:55 pace.

August 25

Another yoga-free yoga day. D'oh.

August 26

Up early to run a five-mile double loop around town. I take the dog with me. She poops at the fire house. I have to carry it with me for a mile and a quarter before I hit a trash can. At least it's not too humid.

On the second loop, a squirrel scolds us from a tree directly over our heads. The dog stops short and stares straight up, frozen solid. I don't know how I don't trip over her. It takes me a couple of tries to drag her past the squirrel.

10:44 per mile, not counting squirrels.

August 27

Up early again, for another five-mile run. This time I decide to run down Sunset Boulevard. It's early enough in the morning that I'll be able to avoid the treacherous car-and-bicycle traffic. It's actually a very lovely road. The wild clematis is starting to bloom, so the air is almost obscenely floral. The 2.5 miles from my house takes me almost to a beach entrance in Cape May.

I'm surprised to see several other runners out this morning, mostly all after I've turned toward Cape May. They are all about twice my age, and all slower. Except, of course, for the one that blazes past me on my return trip down Sunset. He's twice as old AND twice as fast.

Past the Meadows (another important bird-watching destination here), back into a tunnel of tall trees, I pass an older woman out for a morning walk. It's such a peaceful place here, at this time of day. A few moments after I pass her, a large tanker truck comes up past me. The truck is loud and an odd sight coming from Cape May Point. I'm still trying to figure out why he's on the road in the first place when the slightly-disturbed peace of the morning is completely obliterated by a massive BOOOOOM!!!! followed by a short hiss. One of the semi's tires has exploded - right next to the lovely older woman out for her morning walk. The sound is so loud, especially in our tunnel of trees, that I nearly turn around to give the poor woman a hug.

11:28 per mile. The truck is still on the side of the road when we head out for breakfast. The lady is not.

August 28

Time to carbo-load for tomorrow's long run.

Always Make It 13.1

August 29

The training plan says 13 miles, but why go 13 when you could do 13.1? I get up before dawn, enjoy a cup of coffee and an R-bar (ooh, double chocolate!), then hit the road. My legs are not with me for the first mile, and my phone tells me I have just completed a 12:08 mile. This could be a long morning.

Fortunately I wake up a bit as I watch the sun rise up onto a canvas of clouds. It looks like a bad painting. "Not realistic", I think to myself, even though I'm looking right at it.

I hear turkeys gobbling at me from behind some hedges in West Cape May, and two guinea hens cluck at me sleepily. I pull myself up and over the canal bridge. On the other side, a totally adorable couple is heading up. She is running, and he is on a bike. They have matching reflective vests. Too cute. Much cuter than the biking-and-running couple I once saw in Tucson. She had an exhausted look on her face, and he had a handgun in his wasteband. I made up stories in my head about some new extreme-training trend where a guy shoots at your feet if your pace slows. I'll take matching vests over that any day.

On the other side of the canal, there is an oversized dead herring on the road. I stop to take a picture.

Closer to the Ferry Terminal, there is a loose dog on the road. She keeps looking back at me, but then she runs away as if she thinks I'm chasing her. I slow my pace to see if she'll come to me, but she just runs into the phragmities. She's old and has a bit of a limp. Poor thing.

The outward trip takes me into the parking area for the Ferry.   The MV Delaware is loaded up and ready to pull out when I get to the end of the sidewalk. I pause for a moment to enjoy the view, and the horn blows just as I turn to head home. What perfect timing.

The dog is still running along the road when I come back. A car has pulled over to try to catch it, and for that I am thankful. The dog is still unsure of us, though, and won't come near. The lady says she thought she saw a picture of that dog as being missing, so hopefully she can let the owners know where their poor dog is.

The return trip seems like a breeze. When I get back, I realize I have beat my previous half-marathon (of which I have run four official and one just for fun) PR by 2.5 minutes. This is especially miraculous since my previous times have all been pretty consistent, whether I walk for a mile or run the entire time.

Average pace 11:01. New half marathon record: 2:23:27.

August 30

Rest. My left calf, or slightly to the inside of my left calf, is sore.

August 31

My last six-mile run here. I can't believe it's the end of my time in New Jersey already. I savor it and stop to take pictures of some of my favorite sights along my route.   The farm fields, the hidden pathways, the clematis that is starting to resemble unending snowbanks on the sides of the road, and the dozen wild turkeys that dash across the road just before I reach the Canal.

I take an extra minute to soak in the view from the side of the Canal. I can see the Ferry at the terminal. Just before I start to run back, I blow a kiss to the Ferry. It honks back immediately.

10:37 pace. The pictures don't do it justice.

September 1

Yoga day. I'm getting very bad at these.

September 2

Five-mile run around town before it's time to pile into the car and go horseback riding. I get up early. It's foggy. The sunrise is hazy and beautiful over Lighthouse Pond near the State Park. On my second loop around town, the fog has lifted - slightly. It now hangs about eight feet above the ground, like a ghostly ceiling. It is bizarre, to say the least, but also beautiful.

I take full advantage of the fruits of my town. I grab and nibble on Russian olives and beach plums as I pass them. No race refueling station could beat this.

11:04 per mile. I must have stopped too many times for snacks.

Victory Lap in New Jersey

September 3

Last run in New Jersey. I bring the dog along, as it is
also her last run in New Jersey. We make it two doors down
before she has to poop. We're so close to the house, I
double back and toss the poo bag up into the driveway and
start our run again. The rest of it is fairly smooth sailing.
Past the post office, the fire hall, the dunes, Lake Lily,
Lighthouse Pond, the lighthouse, the nun's retreat, my
church, the houses of my friends… I'm going to miss this.

10:44 pace. I kind of wish I'd gone slower and
savored it more.

September 4

A day to rest. Also a day to pack. In the afternoon
we drive up to Philadelphia International to pick up my
husband, then keep going to spend the weekend at our
friends' house in the hills of Pennsylvania. On Sunday they'll
hold the Fatty Burger Fourth of July Feast of Gluttony, a

long-standing tradition that has obviously changed dates over the years. Now that we're all old and have jobs, Labor Day Weekend is a much more feasible time to bring us all together. A few of us have even become runners, so we're planning on holding Fatty Burner, the first (but hopefully not last) annual 5k, on Sunday. But not me; I'll be back watching the kids so that the husband can run; I have to run 10 miles tomorrow.

September 5

I have to run 10 miles today. Due to some miracle, I wake up at 6am. The kids and husband are sleeping next to me on air mattresses. I have left my running clothes in the hall, so I sneak out and grab them, then slink into the bathroom to get dressed. It is here that I realize that I have forgotten underwear. They are in the suitcase in the room where the rest of my family is sleeping. It's too risky. I decide to go without. To add to the irony, I own only one pair of running shorts without an inner underwear-like lining, and it is this one pair that I have packed.

I slip stealthily down the stairs and sit at the kitchen table eating a granola bar while I wait for the sun to come closer to rising. It is cloudy outside, and dark. We are out in the country here, with no street lights and few house lights. It's beautiful, but maybe not optimum for running in the dark. By 6:30, it is light enough to head out. My ninja skills help me open the sliding door and slip out onto the deck in absolute silence. The entire house sleeps peacefully as I come around through the driveway, ready to hit the road. Except, I find out upon returning, for the fact that I tripped their security system on the way through the driveway, so my friends were awoken by a notification email with a photo of a dork in short shorts wandering through their driveway at the buttcrack of dawn. (They forgive me.)

The first two miles of the run take me through rolling farm fields. Corn taller than my head, piles of hay taller than my house, and huge cows that moo as I run by. Pastoral.

At the two mile mark, I cross a semi-busy street (one car) and head up a hill. The huge fields are quickly replaced by massive trees. The hill goes up. And up. And up. I'm starting to regret my decision to come up this beast, but now that I'm on it I can't turn around. I also can't run in a straight line, as a fleet of worms is crossing the road. Thousands upon thousands of worms, wiggling their way from the left side of the street to the right. I'm too much of a hippie to step on any of them, so I jog like a fairy on tip-toes up this crazy hill. My legs are burning. I finally reach the top - 425 feet in one mile - and start coming down the other side. This feels good for a split second before I remember that I'll have to come back up this steeper hill on the way back. I promise myself that I will NOT run up this hill.

At the foot of the hill, I turn left and pass the Boyertown Waterworks. I pause to look at it, knowing that it'll probably be the last water I'll see on a run for quite some time. Turn around, back up the hill. I do walk it, and even walking up this steep hill has me out of breath. On the way back down, I feel like I'm flying. At least, I would feel like I'm flying if I didn't have to look out for these crazy worms. I'm thankful when I cross the "busy" road again (two cars this time) and get back to the worm-free roads that meander through the farms. Back to my friends' house, ready for a weekend of gluttony.

12:07 pace. Respectable, given the hills. And worms.

September 6

Move over day of rest; I'm ready for a week of rest. After telling my friends about how beautiful my route was yesterday, they scratch the plan for a 5k and decide to do the same 10 miles. They get to the top of the hill, start going down the other side, curse me (No no, when I said hill, I meant HILL!), turn around, and come back after just 8 miles. Their average pace is 16 minutes. (They forgive me.)

All my mileage this week will be done in the car. Today we dash down to New Jersey to drop off our borrowed air mattresses, pick up our dogs, and finish packing the car. It's time to drive back to Tucson. We're taking the scenic route, so we won't arrive until a week from today.

High and Dry

September 14

And here we are, back in the desert. After months of running through cool breezes and beautiful scenery, and after a week of sitting in the car and eating burgers and fries, I drag myself over to the YMCA to run 7 miles on a treadmill overlooking a dumpster.

My legs are more ready for this feat than my head. I have to force myself not to look down and check the mileage every second. I think I'm doing well for the first four miles, but then all the road trip catches up to me. I take a moment to walk. At the five-mile mark, I reset the treadmill. It times out after an hour, and it's going to take me much longer than that to get this run done.

I do get it done, though. 11:29 pace. My hips are sore.

September 15

The cure for not actually doing yoga at home: Doing yoga at the YMCA. They just happen to have a class that lands on a Tuesday. I have taken that class on and off (mostly on) for years, so I'm looking forward - mostly - to going back. I say "mostly" because, in my tenure there, they have gone through 11 instructors. Most of them have been good; two of them have been spectacular. The most recent instructor I'd experienced there was a great teacher, but she taught exactly the type of yoga I dislike - Vinyasa. That's where you move constantly, going through various sets of poses like a dance. I dislike this for two reasons. One is that I can barely handle running, where the moves are "left foot, right foot, repeat" for miles and miles. If you so much as tell me to move an arm along with that, I'll get confused and probably fall over. I am not a dancer. The other is that the thing I love most about yoga is that it unties everything I've tightened up with running. My hamstrings, hips, psoas, IT band, shoulders - everything that I'm crunching up with running gets stretched back out, and I return to the trail (or treadmill) feeling refreshed. With Vinyasa, I just about start to hit a good spot and it's time to get right back out of the pose and do the next one (or, in my case, probably fall over). I tell myself that if the awesome Vinyasa instructor is still there, at least it'll be closer to the "cross training" to which my training plan is probably referring, which would be a good thing. No, really. Good.

So off I go to the Y. The yoga classroom (I use the term loosely; it's actually the multi-purpose room, whose walls are peppered with decorations for their after-school program; this is NOT the yoga dome at Canyon Ranch) is half-full when I arrive; it fills up completely within a few minutes. The instructor is someone I don't recognize but whom I instantly like, and whose name I instantly forget (along with "ability to move gracefully", "ability to remember a name for half a second" was not one of the gifts bestowed upon me at birth). After a warmup that feels so good I almost want to cry (My neck pops! My shoulders pop! My back pops! My ankles pop! A lot! I must have increased my volume by 50%), the instructor says we'll be working on hip openers. Now I really do cry (or at least my hips do). This is fantastic. And then, we flow. We flow from one pose to another, barely holding anything for more than half a second. Yup, Vinyasa. At the end of class, my hips feel no better than they did yesterday. The lovely instructor had told us that she teaches "all kinds" of yoga. I am hoping she delves into one (ANY) of the other kinds next week.

This counts as cross training. Good. No, really.

September 16

Back on the treadmill again for six miles. I'm thankful that it's less than the seven miles of two days ago, and excited that I'll be down to five for tomorrow. It's fun when each day is a little easier than the last. We won't think about the fourteen coming up on Saturday.

My pace is slow on the treadmill. I end up walking for a few minutes. I walk not because I am tired or out of breath, but because of a song that pops up on Pandora. "Dark Eyed Molly" - a song written by Archie Fisher and sung by my dear Stan Rogers, but this is a woman singing it. First I have to check if it was, indeed, Archie Fisher who wrote it. It was. For some reason I think I can find an explanation as to why this woman (whose voice was actually lovely) was singing it, but a quick Google search tells me that is not a question anyone had anticipated. I almost feel ready to start running again when we reach the last lines of the song - "I long for his deep, dark eyes". The original line, having been written and sung by men, is "I long for HER deep, dark eyes". Of course a woman singing it would probably change the gender, but the song is still called "Dark Eyed Molly"; is she singing about a man named Molly?

It is stuff like this that keeps me in the left foot-right foot realm. No dancing for me.

I run again when the song is over.

11:37 pace, thanks to my running mind.

September 17

Last day on the treadmill this week. Five miles, hopefully distraction-free. I realize I'm running out of things to write about. When I started the run, my view was of three YMCA vans, a closed gate, a dumpster, and the distant Santa Catalina Mountains. By the time I am finished, the gate is open. This must count for my excitement for this run.

11:12 pace. I managed to up the pace every mile, then every quarter mile for the final one. I own the negative split.

September 18

Rest day. I spend the day drinking water in preparation for tomorrow and trying to remember where I unpacked all my longer-distance running gear.

September 19

Fourteen miles! I've never run this far before. It's back to running along the multi-use paths that run next to the washes (dry river beds that fill with angry brown garbage-filled fast-moving mud-water after storms) that go all around Tucson. They have the benefit of not having to cross a million streets, driveways, business accesses, etc; wherever the path comes to a bridge, it dips conveniently under it. No traffic to worry about. Doubly good in Tucson where I've seen folks driving on the sidewalks for inexplicable reasons on more than one occasion. The drawback is that Tucson has a healthy-sized homeless population, and they frequently sleep under these bridges. And then there are all the reports of sexual assaults along the paths. And the times I've come across drug paraphernalia. And the time there was the person spread out next to all her drug paraphernalia. So it's a battle between avoiding the sidewalk drivers, avoiding the summer sun, and avoiding the running-alone-in-the-dark-and-being-a-target issue. I opt to head out the door right at dawn.

The path is just over a mile from my house. Before I get there, a man walking on the shoulder of a busy street, rather than the sidewalk, crosses for some reason to walk right behind me. I am just about comfortably far from him (I am running faster than he is walking, after all), a man comes out from behind a bush right near me. He is also slow-moving, though. I feel like I'm in an odd don't-get-raped video game. Neither of them are visible by the time I run on the portion of sidewalk where someone has scrawled, "On this spot my 12-year-old daughter was sexually assaulted in 1994" or something to that effect. I can't run and read at the same time, and I've never stopped to look at it. I haven't even gone a mile yet and I want to turn around and go home, but then I'd have to pass through the gauntlet of road-crossers and bush-hiders. I press on.

One mile takes me to Culver's. They are one of the many midwestern/western burger chains (of which there are three within a mile of my house) that have moved into the area. This one touts "butter burgers". No matter how slow I am, they will not be open by my return trip. Lucky them.

Down and onto the running path I go. I am pleased to find that it is already busy with runners, walkers, and cyclists. I loved being the only person on the road in New Jersey, but here I take comfort in numbers.

There is no water in the wash. It is amazingly green, though. Clearly there was a good monsoon (the summer rainy season) for so many plants to be sporting such green leaves. I see a few rabbits. A roadrunner dashes across the path in front of me. I hear quail calling down in the wash. A trio of Cooper's Hawks darts crazily across the path. I duck to avoid having them get caught in my hair.

Time to head under the first bridge. I could tell just by the smell that I am almost there; thousands of bats make this bridge their home, and the stink of guano permeates the air. There had been a small camp up on the side of it, but today I see no sign of it. There is a man on the far side of the bridge. He lives there with his tomato plants. I wonder if he's from New Jersey and he's as tired of the in-ground motor-home style architecture of most of the neighborhoods as I am.

I follow along the wash as far as this trail will take me, but it's not that far. Not quite five miles into my run, the path turns away from the wash and goes up a residential street. I'm far enough away from the main part of town now that I am passing houses with land. These folks have a couple of cows and a small fallow field. Across the street are several horses. It's my favorite part of the run.

The road is short, though, and then I'm running along a fairly busy road. The paved path continues along this road, crosses a wash, and goes up a good little hill next to a quarry. The quarry has been closed for decades, as far as I can tell, but has a sign on the gate: "Back in 5." I don't think so.

At the six-mile mark, which comes later than I thought it would, I walk for a minute and eat an energy gel. It's a banana-peach flavored one. I'd had one handed to me at an aid station during a half marathon a few months ago, and I thought it was fantastic. The one I'm eating now is warm from being in my black pouch against my warm body. It is not fantastic. Not to self: freeze these next time.

I reach the dead end of the running path. Across the street is some construction equipment; they are working on the next portion of the path. It is scheduled to be done a week after I need it. When they had the groundbreaking a few months ago, they found a body that had been there for quite some time. It disturbs me to think of how many times I'd run right past a dead body.

I turn left and am now running on a sidewalk next to a busy road. It's not too bad this early on a Saturday morning, though. I hear a car honk behind me. I turn around, confused, only to see that it's my husband. He and the kids had gone out to the coop to pick up our vegetables, and they have come this way to cheer me on. They are wonderful. They make a u-turn at the next intersection and cheer me on one more time before they head home. So wonderful. Even moreso because I know I'm about to turn around and head home as well. Any time now. Soon. Any time. It takes much longer than I expect for my running app to announce I've gone seven miles. It does, though, and I turn and head back up the hill. It's a little harder than I expected. When I turn back past the quarry, the breeze seems to have stopped. Moments later, the little wispy clouds that had gently veiled the sun have disappeared. I no longer feel good. I stop at a playground to refill my water bottles, and I don't want to move anymore. For the next few miles, the sun plays a taunting game with me. A little light cloud covers it, and I feel like I can run forever. The cloud goes away, and I instantly want to lie down and die. Cloud comes, I am invincible. Sun, raisin. The clouds don't come often enough. I walk a bit.

I get to Culver's, and I know I have exactly one sunny mile left. My running app is slow in telling me so. Very slow. It's a good quarter of a mile past the restaurant by the time the app chimes in that I'm almost home, even though I know for a fact that I turned around at exactly seven miles and that the restaurant is exactly one mile from my house. Now I am hot, cranky, and confused. Also irritated that it keeps telling me my pace is well over 12 minutes per mile, even though I feel like I'm going much faster than that.

I do finally reach my house. I know I have run 14 miles, so I grab my phone to adjust the distance in my running app. It is only then that I realize I'd had it set to "inside" instead of "outside" this whole time. My phone thought I was running on a treadmill and was measuring my distance without the GPS. I look up my turn-around spot on a map, as best as I can figure where it was, and realize I have run well over the 14 miles I'd set out to do. Not sure where I actually turned around, I estimate my pace at 11:57 over 14.5 (or so) miles. I hate the sun.

September 20

A day to rest up from yesterday. Apart from a giant blister on my right big toe, I feel none the worse for wear after yesterday's run. That's a good sign.

Running in Place

September 21

Back on the treadmill for six miles. As much as I usually dread the treadmill, I'm happy to be in the air conditioning and out of the sun. Although it is, ironically, raining today. It's lovely to watch it drizzle into puddles. Nothing is sore except for my left calf, and that's always sore, so I'm happy. I start out slowly, but I up my pace every mile. My sixth mile takes only 9:44. Part of that is because the rain has been upping its pace as well, and I know I need to get home to keep an eye on the dog. She is absolutely terrified of the gentle pitter-patter of rain on the roof and is likely to tear apart my couch (for safety!?) if I don't get home soon.

Six miles at 11:06. Couch is intact.

September 22

Yoga day, and once again I do yoga. I try hard to remember the instructor's name again (It's either Chrissy or

Christy, I'm 85% sure.), and once again she does a lot of flow work but I enjoy it anyway. I wonder if she thinks I'm just slow when I hold a pose for longer than the rest of the class. It wasn't Yin, but my body feels better after the class.

September 23

Six treadmill miles. After a few extra thunderstorms yesterday, the air has dried completely and I can't even watch little clouds over the mountains.

I increase my pace with each mile again. My last mile is 9:42. I take pride in being two seconds faster than Monday.

10:54 pace.

September 24

Five miles seems so much more doable on the treadmill. The treadmill resets at one hour, and it takes me nearly an hour to run five miles. Any time I do more than that, I have to start it back up again. It's like the treadmill knows no human should be stuck on it for such a long time.

11:23 per mile. Increasing the pace at every mile is nicer, too, when you don't have as many miles.

September 25

Rest day, in preparation for my short-long run tomorrow. Just 10 miles to do, so I have a nice plate of pasta and call it a day.

September 26

My second run outside since I got to Tucson. I take the same route as last Saturday. Unlike last Saturday, I remember to set my running app to use the GPS.

Having seen so many people on the trail last week, I leave a little earlier. The sun is just starting to turn the very top of Cathedral Peak in the Santa Catalina Mountains a lovely purple-pink as I head north for a mile. It is a quiet, peaceful time of day.

I remembered my hat this time, too. I haven't quite gone a mile when I notice an inchworm measuring the brim. I stop and let him off at the nearest tree. The sidewalk is overgrown, with just enough space for my feet in the center. I am mindful that there may be rattlesnakes hidden in the grass. Must remember that on the return when the temperature is a bit warmer.

Down on the running path, I head south. There are wet, muddy spots in the wash from the rains this past week. The water had been running for a bit, but this morning there are just a few small puddles tucked into the shadier spots.

I pass a few runners going the other direction. We give the obligatory runner's half-wave.

Ten miles takes me to the cow and back. There is a cow on the short stretch of road that connects the wash trail to the portion of the path that goes past the quarry. I never noticed her until one morning last year when she was mooing so loudly and insistently that I was afraid she was about to jump over her fence and trample me. She is quiet this morning. I smile at her as I turn around. Do cows understand smiles?

There are two drinking fountains along my route, so this morning I did not pack any of my own water. The water in both of them is warm, but it tastes delicious.

Just before I come back up from the wash trail, I see a beautiful Gambel's Quail standing on the side of the wash. Drinking fountains and quail. There are benefits to running here, even if it's getting to be too hot to be outside already at 8:00am.

11:23 average pace. I get home to find my husband weeding the front yard. This is a good day.

September 27

Rest. My calf is very sore, and I have had an inch-wide blister on my big toe for almost two weeks. I have been rotating two pairs of running shoes. They both have nearly 700 miles on them. I have had a brand new pair in my closet, waiting until the time is right. I take them out. The time might just be right. They are identical to one of the pairs I have been running in (I'd found a great deal, so I bought two pairs), so I compare the two. Strangely, the new pair does not have large holes along the sides. The soles are a good quarter inch thicker, and the tread is not half-missing. Perhaps I'll take these for a spin tomorrow.

September 28

Seven miles on the treadmill. I pretend that my new shoes will make this more exciting. The shoes are not the amply-padded epiphany I'd hoped for; my calf is still sore. Still, the miles go quickly. Some of my favorite sea chanties come on, and that helps. There are old men on the treadmills to my left and right. I'm sure they think I'm listening to some noisy rock on my earbuds. I wonder what they'd say if they knew what I really heard.

11:16 per mile. My calf is complaining less at the end than it had in the beginning. When I take my shoes off at home, I notice that my giant blister has popped. I sort of wish I'd taken a picture of it.

September 29

Yoga days really do happen more regularly when there is a class to attend. Today we work on back bends. I snap, crackle, and pop my way through, loving every minute of it.

September 30

My last run this month, six miles. At the end, I am seven miles short of running 100 miles in the month of September. I feel no urge to go on a seven mile run this evening, though.

I do my weekday runs on the treadmill at the YMCA near my house. They have a nice group of people to watch my kids, otherwise I wouldn't be able to do this at all. We go at about the same time every morning so that my kids have the same group of other kids to play with. I also have the same group of folks "upstairs" in the gym around me. Except for a few other moms, I am the youngest there by half. A small posse of old folks roam the Y in the mornings, drinking coffee, gossipping, and occasionally walking on a treadmill for several minutes at a time. They are, each of them, awesome. This morning as I finish wincing my way through my six miles (my left calf was only willing to do 0), one of the old gentlemen materializes next to me and leans his head over toward me. "You're a workhorse, aren't you?!" he says to me. "A real workhorse!" He disappears almost as quickly as he had appeared, off to share some news with his friends, but the smile stays on my face for the rest of my run. Never have I been so happy to have someone call me a horse.

11:31 average pace. I heard of a study once that they had people do identical workouts on treadmills and "in real life", and those on the treadmill thought they had worked much, much harder. I truly understand that study.

October 1

Back on the treadmill. Five miles today. 11:25 per mile, and no one called me a horse. Well, my left calf called me a few things, but I'll not repeat them here. I buy myself a set of arch supports to see if that helps. I know I pronate, and I know I pronate more on my left leg, and it is the inside of that calf that hurts the most, so somehow this makes sense. We'll see if it works.

October 2

Tomorrow I have to run farther than I've ever run before. I need to stop letting that fret me, as I'll be saying it too many times over the next couple of months for it to be a source of stress.

After a carb-filled lunch ("I'll have the side of tots, please"), we drive up to a running store for a packet pick-up. My husband is doing a triathlon tomorrow morning. While we're there, I have the shoe experts measure my feet. I have one and a half black toes, two popped blisters, and an entire set of toes on which I'm never quite sure where the callous ends and the toenail begins. I had stocked up on running shoes when I first started running, after getting a professional fitting at this running store, but I wonder if my feet have changed enough through so much running that I should be wearing something else. After a quick measure, I am told that I am wearing the right brand and style for my foot, although I pronate a bit and could use some arch supports. I promise myself a little gold sticker when I get home. As for the toes? They will just have to deal with it.

October 3

Ah, the trials and tribulations of an active couple. My husband has dibs on the morning, since he has his triathlon. I bring the kids up to cheer him on. He does very well, placing in the top third. I am proud of him, and only a little jealous of his naturally fast-paced running, but I also wish he had gone a bit faster. It is 10:00 by the time we get home, not a cloud in the sky, and the temperature is already creeping above 90.

It's only going to get hotter, so I quickly drench myself in sunscreen and head out the door. I have no plans of trying to run the entire 16 miles I have on my training plan for today. I will GO 16 miles, but it's anyone's guess how much of it will be running.

After the first quarter mile, I know I should not be outside for a long time. I opt to do a several loops around from the YMCA to the running path and back. After the second loop, I realize I have to use the bathroom. There is one just south of the loop I have been taking, so on my third loop I head there. I have gone just over six miles, so I pause to have an energy gel and refill my water bottles with lukewarm water from the drinking fountains. I have about had it with the sun, so I head south for a mile, vowing that this will be my final loop.

I have been running almost the entire time, although slowly. My running app tells me I've been averaging 12-minute miles. My seventh mile is decidedly faster than that when I notice that there is a coyote in the wash. In the middle of the day. I slow to look at him for a moment, and he turns and starts coming toward me. Coyote in the middle of the day coming toward me adds just enough adrenaline to the caffeine and carbs I just slurped down. I zoom along the path as I attempt to calmly consider that rabid animals are hydrophobic, so my freshly-refilled water bottles are better than mace.

Just past the seven-mile mark, I turn back to the north. My friendly coyote is still visible, although he has curled up in a comfortable ball in the middle of the sand. If he's not rabid, he must be crazy; I'm starting to wonder if there's a secret running group in Tucson that runs exclusively through the sewers simply for the shade.

I come back up out of the running trail, past the Culver's, and I realize that I'm too grumpy-hot for the siren smell of their french fries to tempt me at all. It's time to get inside.

I head to the YMCA. After taking a moment to refill my water bottles from their delightfully COLD drinking fountain, I climb onto the treadmill at exactly 10 miles into my run. This is the most decadent time I have ever had on a treadmill. I take the one directly next to the giant floor fan, turn it on full blast, and aim it straight for my head. It feels unspeakably good.

I had been promising myself over the last couple of miles that I was just going to walk once I got to the treadmill, but I find that walking makes my legs hurt. Confused, I crank the speed up to 4.5mph - a dreadfully slow run, but a run no less. This feels better. I spend the next 5.5 miles trying to wrap my brain around the fact that I can run better than I can walk. It is still Linear A when I dismount and jog that final half-mile home.

My average pace 13:14. That is still a running pace, albeit slow as ever. My husband, completely refreshed after his tri, hands me an apple. I am too tired to chew it. My calf feels no more sore than if I had run just six miles. I am happy.

October 4

When I wake up in the morning, I feel no effects at all from yesterday's run. This is a fantastic sign.

October 5

I try to come up with a reason not to do my scheduled 7 miles this morning, but there is none. I'm somewhere between "Just do it" and "Must do it". So I do it.

I work on my pace a bit today. I start out slow, but I up the pace after every mile. This doesn't tire me as much as it had the past few times I'd tried it, so I'm pretty happy. When I'm happy, running feels better. It gets even better when Meat Loaf's "Anything for Love" comes on in the last couple of miles. As dorky as it is, I love running to that song; doubly so since it's so incredibly long I know I'll get at least a mile in before my music-high ends. The seven miles are over before I know it, and I feel great. I can't figure out why my best runs are always the ones I dreaded.

11:07 per mile. After the run, I am treated with a cool, breezy day with fluffy clouds shuffling by. In a daring move, I turn off the air conditioning when I get home.

October 6

Yoga day, except the yoga class is canceled today. The race is exactly two months from today, but I try not to let this worry me. I attempt to stretch a bit, but it's more difficult without anyone there to wrangle the kids for me. In the afternoon we are treated with hail-filled thunderstorms.

October 7

Six miles. I wear my new shoes, but I don't transfer the arch supports over. My feet hurt. My calf hurts. My calf hurts a lot. The pain lessens after a few miles, so I finish strong.

11:00 average pace.

October 8

I have seven miles to do today, but as I walk the distance to the YMCA building from my car in the parking lot, my calf hurts already. I'm nervous that I'm doing damage to it. I understand why runners rely on Dr. Google rather than their real doctors so often; it's easier to ignore it when a website suggests taking a rest (that crazy internet, so filled with wrong information) than when an actual doctor is telling you the same thing. Best to avoid the latter scenario. I've got less than two months left now, after all.

Still, I don't want to really damage my calf, so I do something crazy and head for the elliptical instead of the treadmill. I'll do part of my workout here, then finish up on the treadmill. This seems doubly logical since my leg had started feeling better after it had warmed up just yesterday.

As I get on the elliptical, I think that I haven't been on one since I was pregnant. Within a few minutes, though, memories start flooding back. Specifically, memories of heads creeping into my peripheral vision; the heads of YMCA staff members coming to take me off the elliptical. "Your son is still crying" was the usual scenario. Clearly that was after I was pregnant. The child care folks would take ten minutes to try to calm a crying baby, and after that mom's time was up. My first few months back to working out after having my little mama's boy were filled with 10-minute workouts. After an extended adjustment period, the words of the creeping heads would change a bit. "Your son is attacking other children with Matchbox cars." "Your son pooped and we can't change him." (They wouldn't change cloth diapers, and I didn't feel like going out and buying disposables for those odd occasions when he needed a change.) Maybe part of the reason I switched to running was so that those heads had a little farther to float; the treadmills are past the ellipticals, so I would get an extra seven seconds or so of relaxing sweat-time before I had to go clean up whatever mess my little guy had made this time.

Or maybe it was the nonsensical pacing of an elliptical. I'm not exactly running, I'm not exactly cycling, and I'm not exactly skiing, but it tells me I have covered 2 miles of… road? Snow? Moon rocks? I have no idea. Surely this is not transferable to actual running miles, but it will have to do. My quads are burning. After three miles, I can't feel the fronts of my feet. THAT. That is why I quit the elliptical. Four miles of whatever-it-is, I am done.

I switch over to the treadmill for my last three miles. I am looking forward to it, up until the moment that I actually start the machine up and try to move my legs. They do NOT want to move. I didn't think the elliptical was hard, but my legs are too exhausted to handle this. I slow the pace, but it is still miserable. To top that, my calf actually hurts worse than before I'd started. I slow it down to a walk for a while. I'm feeling better by my third mile, so I start running again. This time it's okay. I up the pace every tenth of a mile. My last mile is less than 10 minutes. I glare at the ellipticals on my way out.

Ever the empath, my son has an accident the moment I get to the child watch to pick him up.

October 9

Rest day.

October 10

A short long run. Just 10 miles. I have to force myself to get out of bed in the morning (so comfy!), but I am rewarded by a cool morning and almost total cloud cover. It's beautiful out. The air smells lightly of creosote, although I don't think we've had any rain overnight. I take the shorter route down to the running path. I'm slow and my calf is sore, but it's just such a nice morning, none of that bothers me. I decided to head north for a mile. There is a roadrunner sitting on top of a rock on the side of the path, puffed up and enjoying the cool morning. When I turn and head south, he is still atop his rock.

I'm starting to recognize people on the trail. There's the self-declared bike patrol man who rides back and forth on the five-mile section of trail. The man with the puffy eyebrows; I'll always remember him because of the time he came out from behind a bush and scared the bejesus out of me. Today he smiles a friendly smile. No ill will. Then there's the nicely dressed old cowboy. He might be a ghost. He looks to be about 80, with a real cowboy hat, and clothes from the 60's that look as if they are brand new. The recumbent bike posse; there are four or five in that group. They always look like they are just about to tell a great joke. I love them. The regular cyclists always seem so irritated at them.

My southbound route takes me past a few rabbits and many flocks of small, unidentifiable birds. Back home today, folks are taking part in the Big Sit. They found a spot to sit at midnight, and there they will stay until midnight tonight, counting how many different species of birds they see in that time. There are multiple teams taking part in this event, each trying to see the largest variety of birds. I'm sure I'm passing some interesting things, and I would enjoy the excuse to sit still for 24 hours…

Back to my run. The clouds are still giving me a treat as I turn back for home. There is no water in the wash, but I can tell by the large portion of car that has arrived in the sandy center that there had been a good flow with Tuesday's storms. The storms also gave the desert a good cleaning; the leaves that are usually dust-covered are looking delightfully green.

I come up out of the running trail and back onto the sidewalk. Today I run up my big hill - a steep but short incline that leads up to my neighborhood. I had been taking a different route partly to avoid this hill, but today it doesn't seem so bad.

My average pace was 11:51. Perhaps I was doing a little too much sightseeing.

October 11, 2015

Rest day. I pretend to be a monkey-lumberjack and swing from some overgrown trees in my yard with a saw. Falling would be bad for my training. I do not.

My sister-in-law, meanwhile, runs the Chicago Marathon today. It's not her first marathon, nor even her first time doing Chicago. What makes this day amazing is that she has been injured for nearly a year and is running it with essentially no training. Her longest training run was over a month ago, and it was only eight miles. Today she does 26.2. I won't tell you how long it took her, because that's not the point. The point is, she did it. With continuing pain and no training, she did not stop moving until she found that finish line. If that's not inspirational, I don't know what is.

October 12, 2015

Seven miles. For my run on Saturday, I was supposed to do "miles 3-5 at marathon pace". This essentially broke my brain. First, I didn't know if they meant my third through fifth miles (so, starting when my app said "two miles"), or starting when I had reached three miles. Surely this makes no difference as far as training goes, but it bothered me that I wasn't sure exactly when to do it. The second half of that assignment was no less confusing as the first. What is my marathon pace? How does one figure that out? I am slow. I will be slow at the marathon. Is there a difference in slowness? There's how fast I would like to be if I ran an ideal marathon (under 5 hours would make me a happy camper), but I have no idea if that's realistic. I'm guessing I'll finish in 5:15 or so. So which pace would I pick? The one that gets me what I want? Or the one I am more likely to have? Or the one that, unbeknownst to my training plan, would give my sore calf the most rest for today?

I finally decided on something in the middle. I think my goal was a slightly more than 11 minutes per mile. That opened the second issue of, how in blazes do I figure out how fast I am running as I am running it? I often feel like I'm running fast only to find that I'm running like a slug, and vice versa. I did realize, though, that my running app gives relatively accurate current speed, so when the pleasant voice announced that I had completed two miles, I pulled it out of my running belt and proceeded to try to up my pace slightly (it said I had been averaging 12:30) and watch my current pace, while (and at the same time) not falling over or running into any hapless folks out for a pleasant morning walk.

It took me all of 1/10 mile to realize this was impossible.

I made up for that on the treadmill today. At the end of two miles, I bumped the speed up from my slow warm-up jog to 5.4 miles per hour (speed demon that I am). I kept it there for three miles. Much easier than trying to figure it out in real life. Score one for the treadmill. I am tempted to say I guessed right, as I found myself so ensconced in my own daydream that I practically forgot that I was running; my legs just DID it. Or maybe it was just a quality daydream. Something along the lines of befriending Paul McCartney, traveling with him to Liverpool to play a joke on my dear old friend from high school, and probably getting to ride his horses a bit as well.

At the end of my "marathon pace", I slow down to my usual warm-up pace for a mile, then gun it up to 6 (a 10-minute mile; the gateway to the single digits!) for the last full mile. I feel great. One of those odd runs where I actually like running WHILE I AM DOING IT. Usually it's more like the classic "banging my head against a wall" ("Why are you doing that?" "Because it feels good when I stop.") act.

11:20 per mile. I enter that into a race pace calculator when I get home. It tells me I will finish in 297 hours. I realize I had put the "11" under "hours" per mile (why do they even have that?), put it in correctly, and it comes back with 4 hours 57 minutes. Wouldn't that be lovely…

October 13

Yoga day, except the yoga class is canceled again today. I put on my yoga clothes anyway, with the hope that I will get around to doing some yoga at home. That doesn't happen.

October 14

Six miles on the treadmill. I appreciate weeks when the treadmill miles decrease as the week goes on. 11:46 pace.

October 15

Five miles to do today. I watch lizards dash back and forth on the ground outside the window. 11:35 pace.

October 16

A day to rest up for my long run tomorrow. It's also my birthday tomorrow, so I am treated to a massage from a friend who is a massage therapist at a posh resort in town. The resort is too posh to let little people like me come in, so she does me in her living room. It feels fantastic. She works hard on that tricky left calf of mine. I can feel all sorts of weird things moving around in there. She tells me I have some "interesting spots" in there. Yup. On the way home, it feels like my leg is getting continuously longer. It doesn't hurt for the entire rest of the day.

October 17

Seventeen miles today. I sleep poorly overnight; we have some lovely loud thunderstorms roll through, so the dog keeps me up. She keeps trying to move pillows back and forth on the floor. It is not supposed to be hot, so I do not even set an alarm. I roll out of bed at a little after 6:15, and I relax on the couch with a decadent cup of coffee.

It is still cloudy when I head out the door. The storms are just moving off. I head north to start, and I can see lightning flashing over the Catalina Mountains. That storm is moving away, so I am safe. I get almost a mile away from my house, and my phone announces I have run a mile. No, I haven't. I have, however, forgotten to tell the phone that I am running outside and not on a treadmill. I pause to reset my run, then turn away from the storm and go down toward the wash. There is just a trickle of water in the wash, but it smells wonderful. Damp dust and creosote.

There is no one out on the trail today. I come upon a set of signs that read something along the lines of "If a dog gives chase/ You better run fast/ If he catches you/ He'll bite your / tire." There is a man associated with these signs, setting up a table full of maps and information about The Loop, the paved multi-use trail that follows many of the washes around town. The city is working on linking them all to make a continuous loop (hence the name) around town. I head over to his table to chat with him for a moment; he seems thankful to have someone visit him.

Up the trail I go. The miles seem to go by quickly. I am not wearing my headphones or even listening to music at all; there are storms popping up all around and I want to be able to hear the thunder if it comes to that. It feels strange going without music, but I do have some playing naturally in my head. Bob Seger is singing "Night Moves" for me. I don't even like that song. But, I did wake last night to the sound of thunder, so there the song sits, stuck on infinite repeat on my mental playlist.

The clouds start to look more forbidding. It starts to smell wetter, and two ducks fly past. Ducks, in the desert. This is probably not a good sign. I run past a coyote. The coyote is trotting along in the wash, looking perturbed. I worry that he feels the pressure dropping and I'm about to get struck by lightning, but instead I am pelted by wind. It starts to pick up, and it just keeps picking up. There is a storm to the southeast, and this must be the outflow from that storm. I check; it is blowing 20mph right in my face. Nothing to do but lean forward and laugh at my luck.

Today is also my grandfather's birthday, or at least it would be had he not passed five years ago. I am reminded of this as I look up at some broken clouds to the east and see a glowing shaft of light dropping from the sky. I pause and take a picture with my phone. I pop my phone back into my waste pack and start running again. I know I am not quite four miles from the spot where I had reset my run, but my running app suddenly announces that I have just completed four miles. Then it tells me I have completed five miles. Then six miles. Then seven. Not bad for just a few moments of jogging. I pull my phone out and look, and sure enough the mileage has bumped up suddenly. I wonder for a moment if the extra miles were a birthday gift from my grandfather. But no, he would never have given me free miles. He would make me earn every single one. I giggle, put my now-behaving phone back into my wastepack, and keep moving.

The wind is intense. I run past some horse pastures, and the sand blows and stings my legs. The trail takes me up and over a slight hill. Ants are walking across the path. The wind is so strong, some of the ants get blown off the ground and fly past me. I have never seen this happen before.

Storms are building up all around me. There are giant shafts of rain falling to the south now. It is beautiful. The rainstorms look like big jellyfish floating across the desert. I reach my halfway point and start to head home. I notice some lightning to the west, but it is far enough that I think it will not reach me. A few raindrops fall on me, but not enough to get me wet. A rainstorm passes north of me. I feel like I'm dodging the jellyfish, but the wind has died down to a much more bearable breeze.

I come to a playground. My husband has brought the kids to the playground so that he can give me some sports drink. I have had two energy gels, and I don't really like sports drinks, but I guzzle some anyway. It makes my stomach hurt and my mouth feel disgusting. I end up drinking the rest of my water just to get the sports drink flavor out of my mouth. Irony.

Just four miles left after my personalized pit stop. The path is now soaking wet after the rainstorm. There is some running water crossing the path, and I have no choice but to run through it. My feet are wet now. They squinch with every step.

As I loop back and start my last mile, my husband drives by with the kids. They are coming from the opposite direction than they should be. The playground is south, but they are coming from the north. The Starbucks is to the north. I spend the last mile hoping that is why they are coming from the north.

I am not disappointed. My husband meets me in the driveway with a frappuccino the size of my head. This is love.

After doing some adjustments, my running app tells me my average pace is 12:01. It also gives me a congratulations for running my fastest mile: eight seconds. Beat that.

October 18
Recovery day.

October 19

Seven miles on the treadmill. My leg is back to being sore, but after my long run Saturday I can't be surprised.

The friendly man who called me a horse a few weeks back pops over again to ask how far I am running. He is very impressed when I tell him. I explain that I'm running my first marathon in December. He tells me I'll do fine; the other runners will be dropping like flies and I'll just keep plugging along. He is sweet.

11:30 per mile. No eight-second miles this time.

October 20

Yoga class is not canceled, but I can't motivate myself to get out the door. While class itself is nice, it's hard to convince myself to get the kids pottied, shoed, car-seated, de-car-seated, walked to the door, brought to the child care area, just for a yoga class that s only slightly what I want. I have access to yoga videos at home, so I opt for one of them. Why, the one entitled "Yin Yoga for Runners" sounds right up my alley, doesn't it? I clear the coffee table away, set up my mat, give it a good spray (holding a pose with my nose to the mat for five minutes is more pleasant when I'm not inhaling feet the whole time), and get started. I make it almost 10 minutes before the kids start doing yoga with me. At first, my six-year-old daughter just sets up her mat next to mine and starts her own routine. Soon her routine starts to creep onto my mat. Next my three-year-old attempts to set up his mat on the other side of mine - in the two-inch-wide space between my mat and the couch. He is, of course, unsuccessful. Deep breaths. Allow myself to sink deeper into the pose. Don't let the yoga mat and half a three-year-old on top of me cause stress.

I explain to them that they should probably move their mats to the more open sections of floor, and that it hurts when they, say, take flying leaps onto my back while I am in Pigeon (which has happened before). My daughter takes the cue and runs off. Moments later, when I'm in half butterfly, she materializes above me and starts working a foam roller up and down on my back. I adore her.

I make it through the hour-long practice, complete with my traditional Savasana under a blanket (substituting "two pretending-to-be-asleep children" for "blanket"). My body feels much better. Yin yoga is awesome.

October 21

I don't know why six miles seems like so much less than seven. Six miles on the treadmill seems like an impressive feat. Seven feels like an act of desperation. I breeze through my run today. 11:11 pace. My calf isn't even that sore. But, my foot doesn't feel good. Hrm.

October 22

Yup, my foot doesn't feel good. It hurts to just walk up and down the hallway. I have seven miles scheduled today, so I get us to the YMCA. It is clear that I should not be running seven miles today. I reason with myself that I have an actual race this weekend, a half marathon, so had I been training specifically for that (rather than just doing it for kicks on a low-mileage weekend; I feel so hard-core!), this would have been a taper week and I would not have a seven mile run on my calendar today. Yes, let's go with that idea. I do hop on for a mile, and by the end of that mile I my foot feels a bit better. It's an 11:28 mile. I am pleased that my body feels warmed up so quickly.

Still wanting to be careful, I switch over to a recumbent bicycle. The typical thing one is told to do with an injury is RICE - Rest, Ice, Compression, and Elevation. I figure a recumbent bike counts as the R and E. Rest, because I'm not actually running, and Elevation, because my foot is up higher than on a regular bike. Right? Right? Yeah, I don't believe myself either. Still, I ride on. I do six miles while reading a book, because I can actually read books while cycling. This is the only benefit I can find. My foot is still sore as I go down to pick up my kids.

October 23

Doctor Google to the rescue. I have extensor tendonitis. Well, I suppose Doctor Google is not quite performing a "rescue" here. Just helps to have a name for the pain I feel. "I have extensor tendonitis" sounds so much less whiny than "My foot hurts." I vacillate between trying to stretch it a bit more so that it doesn't tear more, and trying hard to NOT stretch it a bit more so that it doesn't tear more.

That, and wiggling my toes excruciatingly up and down the way one chews a canker sore.

October 24

A Saturday. This would usually be a day for my long run, but the half marathon I have signed up for is tomorrow. A second day to rest my foot. Score! I rest my foot by walking in flip-flops all around the pumpkin festival so my kids can experience the joys of bouncy pillows, corn mazes, tractor rides, narrow-gauge train rides, and all the other things to make us Tucsonans forget that it's 85 degrees outside and too hot for the actual pumpkin picking act to feel right. We come home with a pair of lovely pumpkins, though, ready to have their innards removed and frightening faces carved into them. We also come home with a foot that feels like a pumpkin. Walking around the pumpkin patch hurt my foot much more than miles I've run after it started to act up.

On our way home, I stop in at a store to pick up my race bib for tomorrow. I am clearly limping my way to the table. The runners manning the table note this. "Extensor tendonitis," I explain. See? Much better than "My foot hurts." They tell me I should run the 5k instead and take some time off. I tell them I have two halves and a full in the next month or so, then I promise to play dead until next year. They nod. It's a runner thing.

Half-Bad Half-Marathon

October 25

Race day! Well, half marathon race day, at least. I sleep fitfully the night before, dreaming repeatedly about the race. It's the naked-at-school dreams all over again, except now it's can't-find-a-parking-spot, showing-up-late, going-off-course, forgot-my-sneakers dreams now. Or the dreams that I have dressed, gone to the race, run the whole thing, and am about to cross the finish line (PR!) just as I wake up to the sound of my alarm telling me I haven't completed a single one of those tasks yet.

My nightly pre-race ritual is to start my french press coffee brewing. I roll out of bed, get dressed, and pop my coffee into the microwave. Whereas in the past, my half marathon breakfast items were carefully pre-planned, this morning I just grab a bowl of cereal.

This race begins in downtown Tucson. As such, there is no specific parking lot. There is plenty of parking - on the streets. My foot hurts, my cheer squad will not be at the finish line, and my running partners are all doing the 5k, I'm not actually sure where the start line is, there's a huge hill in this race and I haven't really run a big hill in a long time, but out of all this, it is the parking that stresses me the most. The last time I parallel parked, I have to admit I did it like a rock star. I also have to admit that was for my driver's test, exactly 20 years ago. I drive through the still-dark morning to the empty streets of downtown Tucson and circle for ten minutes until I find a spot I can just pull into without having to parallel park. My blood pressure instantly drops to a bearable level. Nothing left to stress about today. Except finding the start line.

Luckily, there are vehicles all around with short-shorted folk such as myself climbing groggily out, fiddling with their running belts and safety pins. I follow them. Tucson has an amazingly poorly lit downtown, but soon the sound of music tells me I am following the right people. The party has already started at the start/finish area. I pick up my timing chip (the type you twist-tie to your shoe), then make for the KT Tape tent. Except the tent isn't there. That crazy tent, with the wonderful professionals who love to apply their magical tape to your owie areas, the one that I've noticed before every one of my pain-free races - is not at this one. We have this tape at home, of course, and my husband even tried to give it to me this morning, but I declined so that I could go to the tape tent at the race. My planning was poor. But, I parked! So I switch gears easily. I will run in pain. No problem. Like I said, I parked. Today is a good day.

I find one of my friends and chat with her, up until the moment I realize the race is about to start and I'm nowhere near the start line. So, that dream almost just came true. I do make it to the start line, find a good spot toward the back, and have a good pep-talk with my foot. We will do this.

The race starts late, but these races always do. We do a loop around the library downtown. I am halfway through my first loop when the front of the pack starts zipping past on their second loop. My friend Chad zooms past at a million miles an hour, but he is still somehow able to recognize me from behind and say hi as he zooms. Show off. I find out later that he actually got up at 3am and ran the course once already, for absolutely no reason. Show off.

I am in a nice group of runners, holding a steady pace. The course takes us on an eastern loop after the library. It is basically the 5k that my friends will do later this morning. On the return part of that, I see that there is a man down. An ambulance is already there. EMT's are surrounding him. One of them is on his knees.

They are pumping his chest.

They are blowing air into his lungs. I see his chest rise to an unnatural height, then fall again.

They pump his chest some more.

I keep up my pace. I try not to cry. This man is dead. They are trying to get him back, and God willing, they will, but right now he is dead. A fellow runner, doing what we love, down.

When I get back through the downtown area, my sister-in-law is there to cheer me on. I tell her to pray for the man, and wish her good luck on her race.

We come out of downtown again, past an area where, many years ago, I went on a photography field trip with some of my hiking guide friends. It is bizarre to be here again. We go under I-10, again a bizarre experience, and then up and across a bridge over the Santa Cruz River (which, in the typical style of southwestern rivers, does not actually have water in it). The miles are going quickly now. My foot does hurt with every step, but it's a very bearable pain. I am actually having fun. We start rolling into the Tucson Mountains, and finally we hit The Hill. It's called A Mountain because there is a large A made of painted stones on it, in honor of the University of Arizona. It is uphill. JUST uphill. I turn to start up the hill, as the fast runners are already passing me on their way down.

Suddenly everyone ahead starts to yell. There is a car on the course. A car tearing down the street, right in the middle of all the runners. It's a narrow street, and he's going at least 50. It's a trashy old Pontiac. I have already moved well out of the way as it passes me. The driver, a young man who has clearly already thrown his life away, is smiling at his own daring moves. I pray that he doesn't hit any other folks behind me. A moment later, a police car comes down after him. We all clap loudly for the officer who is giving chase as carefully as he can possibly manage.

Back to the hill. I reach the six mile mark midway up, and six miles is my traditional time to have an energy gel. I have to walk to get it out of my pack, open it, and eat it. This is a welcome break. I find a lucky trash can a few minutes later, so I don't have to carry the sticky trash very far. Double win. Back to running. I am actually not even very tired. I seem to have found the perfect uphill pace. I check my splits when I get home; I ran a 13'57 mile between miles six and seven. Slow, yes, but I also gained 327 feet in elevation.

The view is glorious. When we reach the top, I stop and take a picture.

Down the other side. I find that my foot hurts more on the downhill steps, so I don't take full advantage of gravity on the way down. My downhill pace ends up being the same as my flat pace. Imagine that.

The return route takes us along another part of The Loop. This part goes along the Santa Cruz River. The path here looks just like the portion by my house. More homeless folks sleeping under the bridges here, though. I wonder what they think about 600 runners going by.

Up out of the river, and we are almost home. The last mile is irritatingly uphill. Not steep; just enough to be more winded and less eager to kick than I had hoped. I can't see the finish line until the last minute. It was a beautiful surprise. I dash across; the clock is just turning 2:33:00 as I cross. Later I see that my official time is 2:32:06. I am terribly consistent with my times. It doesn't matter if it's rolling hills, downhill the whole way, one big hill, or even if I run or run/walk; I finish half marathons within 2 minutes of 2:30:00.

I get the medal. I love the medals more than I should. It's just a "certificate of participation", and I bought it with my own money when I signed up for it - but it's so shiny!

I refill my water at the water station. I did a hippie run this time - I had my two clip-on water bottles, so instead of taking paper cups every few miles, I just sipped my own whenever I passed a water stop. I also take a chocolate Muscle Milk; it's the most delicious (official sponsor) chocolate milk I have ever tasted.

I have no idea where I parked my car. No, wait, I do! It was next to the Etherton Gallery. I remember this because it's the only place I ever went downtown before having kids (after which I added "Children's Museum"). I have to look up on my phone where the Etherton Gallery actually is. I find my car. I pull out and find that it's not quite half a block from the Children's Museum. Apparently my downtown parking is as consistent as my half marathon times.

I check the race organizer's Facebook page obsessively after I get home in search of updates on the man who was down on the course, and also out of curiosity on the Pontiac lunatic. I finally hear good news on both fronts; they were able to revive the man, and the police did catch the crazy driver. See? I parked. Today really was a good day.

October 26

I'm trying to reconcile my "I ran a half marathon yesterday" tradition of doing simple yoga with my "I am training for a full marathon" plan of a six mile run. Not to mention the desperate attempt to reconcile my urge to rest my foot with my urge to stick to the plan and not lose any training ground. I choose poorly on both fronts, strap on my sneakers, and head to the gym. I run a full 0.05 miles before I realize just how poor a choice this was. The pain is unbearable. I get off and head toward the recumbent bike again (half a RICE!), but there are four people (somehow) on the three recumbent bikes at the gym. I head for regular bicycle. I really hate the regular bicycle. The miles go fast, yes, but the minutes go slowly. This one has a seat like a rubberized beach cruiser. I have the option of sitting up (Oh! My ischial tuberosities!) or leaning forward (well, that's a slimy handlebar). I go back and forth between the two. I hate them both. My foot doesn't hurt as much as running, but I still feel it with every turn. I manage five miles.

Whatever workout I missed in the gym this morning, I more than make up for it at home, stressing about my foot. My foot hurts. Whine.

Initiate Panic Mode

October 27

Yoga day. At least I don't have to stress over whether to skip a run today or not. I do the Yin Yoga for Runners video again. It feels great. But my foot still hurts.

October 28

Really, my foot hurts. I look at my training schedule. I have 18 miles to run on Saturday. Can I do that if my foot hurts? Should I do that if my foot hurts? If I run today, I will be in better shape for my 18 miles. If I run today, I am more likely to make my foot worse so that I can't do my 18 miles. I try to listen to the advice of most of my running friends and the billion articles I've read on the Internet, and I skip the gym. It does not feel great.

To help myself feel better, I look at the week before my marathon. Just a few very short runs, then I will do the 26.2. If I can do short runs and then run a marathon that week, I can skip a longish run and do 18 miles this week.

I am cranky the whole day. I have been cranky for the past few days. Part of it is probably the stress over running versus not. I suspect part of it is that I am missing the endorphins I collect during my runs. I'm not usually one to get stressed out, or to get grumpy because of stress, but these past few days I've felt like my brain just doesn't want to be happy. I had joked before that I liked to run because it feels good when I stop; I'm starting to think it really DOES feel good when I stop. Just not when I stop this much. I vow that I will run the five miles on my schedule tomorrow.

October 29

Today is the day I had vowed to run five miles. Today is also the day the thunder decided to rumble in the morning. My dog is freaking out. Now I'm freaking out. Should I take the thunder as a sign that I should not run today? Can I still do 18 miles if I skip today entirely? And what about the fact that I'm out of milk? (Not actually related, but I had planned to go shopping after the gym, and the dog barometer is making this challenging.)

There is no storm heading toward our house. The thunder we hear is passing well to our south. I look at the radar obsessively. Nothing is coming our way. As soon as the dog calms down, we rush out the door to the YMCA. I do run five miles. It feels fantastic. My foot is tight but not painful, and I even feel a little pain in my calf. This is somehow a good thing. My foot had been so sore, it had masked the always-there pain in my calf. My calf usually warms up and stops hurting after a few miles, so I keep moving.

What is not a good thing is the way the sky outside suddenly gets dark again. I see the raindrops. Warnings start to pop up on my phone that lightning has struck near my location and I should seek shelter. I look at the radar; a storm has built up from absolutely nothing to a big red storm right over my house. I still have a mile or two left, but I calculate the time it would take me to stop, go get the kids, get them to the car, and drive home. It's just a half a mile between my house and the Y, but it will take a good 20 minutes if I leave right now. In 20 minutes, the storm will be gone. The dog has surely already done whatever damage she will do. I keep running.

11:11 pace. And yes, we go buy milk. The sheets have been removed from my bed, and there is a nugget of poo in the middle of the living room, but the house is otherwise in one piece. As is my foot.

October 30

Rest day. I take it easy on my foot.

October 31

It's Halloween, but I am not afraid of the 18 miles. I get a late start, but the weather is pleasantly cool. I even make a last-minute wardrobe change from my short shorts to capris. For once, I remember to set my running app to "outside" from the start. And off I go…

I am slow. I can't make my legs go. By the time I turn around, my legs are tired. By the time I hit mile 13, my body is TIRED. I am tempted to walk, but I realize that walking hurts my foot much more than running. So I keep running. I am trying not to worry about how exhausted I feel on this measly 18 mile run, and what a bad sign that is for me doing a whole marathon. Nope. Not gonna think about that.

My last mile is slightly uphill for the first half, and I am thirsty, so I walk for a good while as I drink the last of my water. My foot feels tight and sore. When I turn for the last third of a mile to my house, a tiny bit of a downhill, I start running again. It feels surprisingly good! When I was walking, I was highly aware of every part of my body that was sore. Now that I'm running again, I feel refreshed! My mood instantly switches from doom to relief.

My pace was as slow as I felt - 12:38 per mile average. My fastest mile was 11:44 - 14 seconds slower than my AVERAGE pace at the half marathon last weekend. Did I not eat well? Did I not hydrate enough? Was it the runs I skipped this week? I vow to take better care of myself. I ice my foot before I even take a shower. I ice it a few more times throughout the day. It does not feel bad.

November 1

I am relieved to find that I'm not sore today. My foot has sensation but not pain. I ice it a few times today. There will be no runs skipped in the upcoming week.

November 2

Six miles on the schedule turn into six miles in reality. I even crank the pace back up a bit. 11:06 average pace. I don't get to ice my foot until after the kids are in bed. Better late than never.

November 3

Yin Yoga for Runners. Relaxing and useful.

November 4

Five miles today. It feels good to be back on schedule, after my not-even-a-week off. My pace shows it: 10:57 per mile average. When was the last time I dipped below 11 minutes?

November 5

Six miles today, and it still feels good. I admit I'm just as excited to have two days in a row off after this, but that knowledge just makes this run feel even better. 11:16 per mile.

November 6

Rest day. I am being good and icing my foot, even if it's just one time a day. Marathon Day is one month from today. I can't decide if I am explodingly excited or if I literally can't believe that I am actually going to run a marathon a month from today.

November 7

Extra rest day. The schedule calls for a 13-mile run today, but I am signed up for a half marathon tomorrow. Nothing to do but rest. And go on a short hike with my kids, but that still counts as rest. We go to Bear Canyon, and we sit next to the actually-flowing water and nibble leftover Halloween candy. This is the life.

Second Half

November 8

Race Day. Well, half race day. Half marathon day. This one starts from a local high school (my husband's alma mater, as a matter of fact), and as such it has its own parking lot. Stress levels are low. I leave early enough to get a good parking spot, then relax in my warm car (it's 50 degrees outside, or "cold" by Tucson standards) as I watch teenagers attempt hilariously to count the number of cars in the lot and wave the clogged river of incoming traffic toward the empty spaces.

I decide to make a break for the bathroom while the lines are short. On my way out, I run into a friend with whom I have run several times. I wasn't expecting to see her; she usually does overnight runs, ultramarathons, and other such eccentric things. It's nice to see a friendly face. She jokes that she had to reset her mind to doing a "normal" race. I tell her we'll do the American River 50-Miler (a race on which I have my heart set, despite not even having completed a marathon yet) together soon.

I pop back to my car to get my bib on, drop off my jacket, and get my pre-race snack. They have free coffee, so I blow the minds of all around me when I take a half cup of coffee and empty a chocolate-flavored goo into it. It is delicious. They are jealous.

The starting line is on the track of the high school, and they announce that stretches are being led on the 50-yard line. I figure that's not a bad idea, so I head in that direction. Instead of stretching, though, I run into my sister-in-law (who is running the 5-k that starts just after the half) and my ultra-running friend and their spouses. We end up chatting until it's time to line up, and I don't stretch a thing.

I ran this race last year. It was my second half marathon, but the first time I had RUN 13 miles. I remember turning the corner on the track to hit the finish line, knowing that I hadn't walked at all and was sure to have shaved time off of my previous record, only to see that I had added a full minute to my time. I had somehow managed to run slower than I walked. 2:30:50. This year, however, the race organizers had brought in pacers. Since I seemingly always finish half marathons within 75 seconds of 2:30:00, whether I walk, run, have a huge hill to climb, or that one time when I got trapped in a port-a-potty, my natural tendency was to head to the 2:30:00 pacer. I don't. I go to the man holding the sign that says 2:15.

The race starts. The 2:15 pacer is holding a comfortable pace. He explains to some of the people chatting with him that we'll take an easy pace to start, then speed it up a bit toward the end. Much better than starting too fast and tiring out with too many miles left. The pace we are doing, however, is the top of what I want to do. I don't imagine that I'll keep it up for long, and I know I will not want to speed up at the end. Still, I can do it now, so I do it now.

The pacer grabs water at every stop and drinks it - without walking. I have no idea how anyone can do that. I have my water bottles, with their squirt tops, and I still need to walk to drink it.

I keep up with the pacer for much longer than I had expected. It isn't until a very long uphill at mile 10 that I start to lose sight of him. It is a hill that we had just gone down, turned around at the bottom, then back up again. When I am almost to the top, and have almost lost sight of Mr. 2:15, I notice the 2:30 pacer going down the hill on the other side of the road. Yes, I am losing the 2:15 group, but "my" group hasn't even gone down the hill yet. I can slow down. I am doing just fine.

My legs are tired enough that the last three miles are less fun than the first 10, but I'm okay. I hurdle two dead rattlesnakes, high-five some random strangers on the side of the course, then head back toward the school to the finish line. To reach the finish line, one must pass all the faster runners heading back to their cars. It is a bit disconcerting. Back onto the track, however, volunteers are there to hand me a little American flag. This is, of course, a Veteran's Day race. I wave the flag proudly as I turn the corner and see the clock - 2:13:30! And next to me, eating a banana on the sidelines, is the 2:15 pacer - he's not even walking back to his car yet! But wait - why is the 2:15 pacer chilling with a snack when it's not 2:15 yet? As I cross the finish line, I remember that the 5k started five minutes after the half marathon, so they had reset the finish line clock. I don't even care. In my mind, 2:13 is the same as 2:18. I have ROCKED this race. Twelve minutes off my time from the previous year. My running app tells me I did it in 2:15:55 (I believe the official time), at a 10'29" average pace. My slowest mile today was my average pace on the half marathon two weeks ago.

My cheering crew is at church again. I grab a banana, guzzle my water, and wander back to my car. I pass Mr. 2:15 on the way.   I tell him thanks.

November 9

My muscles feel a bit weary from yesterday, and my foot is less than happy. All this training is adding up, and not always in a good way. I don't even joke with myself that I'm going to do the six miles on my schedule for today. Not running, at least. I do go to the YMCA, and I do go six miles - on the recumbent bike. I realize, of course, that six miles on a bike is nowhere near the same output as six miles running, but I do so hate bikes. Six miles is enough.

November 10

Time to do some yoga. Yoga from home again. I opt for a different yoga video, but still one that says it's for runners. It is a more active practice, with a lot of chest opening exercises. I miss the relaxing stretch of Yin, but at the end I feel like my lungs are huge. I must remember this.

November 11

I am ready to run again. Six miles. My schedule this week is 6-6-6, and Friday is the 13th. Thank goodness I'm not superstitious.

The treadmill is uneventful. It's cold outside, so I wear long pants. This decision is instantly regretted once I get into the heated gym. I challenge myself by not turning the fan on. I am so hardcore. And sweaty.

The schedule tells me to run the middle miles at my marathon pace. I up this from my previous choice of 11'10" per mile to 10'42" because maybe - just maybe - I can. I end up with an 11'00" average pace overall.

November 12

Six miles at an easy pace. 11'25" average.

November 13

Rest day for my 20-miler tomorrow. This will be my longest run yet. All the other long runs felt like I had reached some wonderful goal. Twenty doesn't sound like a wonderful goal. Twenty sounds like I have crossed the threshhold into insanity.

I work to carbo load in preparation. I have actually been doing that all week. On Sunday I made an apple cake. I have been eating that instead of Halloween candy after lunch every day. Yes, that doesn't sound like a real feat, but it is. I hate cake, and I'm not a fan of apples. It is a big deal for me to give up few pieces of scrumptious chocolate and eat a hunk of cake (with no icing! The horror!) instead. Well, no one said training would be easy.

I have a big stack of pancakes for breakfast and a heap of potato salad for lunch. Dinner is a light bowl of homemade borscht. I must remember not to stress if anything red comes out of me tomorrow.

One of the folks from the running group that put on the marathon a few weeks ago sends out an email filled with good news. The man who had gone into cardiac arrest is doing well, and may even be able to run again in the semi-near future. The lunatic in the Pontiac, an apparent drunk driver, was arrested and put into jail soon after we all "met" him. All is well that ends well. Take that, Friday the 13th.

November 14

Twenty miles today. Insane. Since the weather is still relatively nice, I sleep in until the kids wake me. I relax and have a cup of coffee and a bowl of cereal. I remember that I haven't clipped my nails, so I do that. It is by far the most time-consuming task of the morning. My runner's toes are thick and confusing, but only one is currently black. I once passed a sign during a half marathon that said something along the lines of, "The God of Lost Toenails smiles on your activity." Too true.

It is just past 7:30 when I hit the road. It is freezing. Well, 52. I am wearing my short shorts and a light shirt, so I am uncomfortably cold for the first mile or so. Being too cold for one mile out of twenty is not bad.

Things are going smoothly all the way until mile two, when I reach up to tighten my pony tail. I have thick, waist-length hair that is delightful when it's a bit cool outside, but is a horrendous heater on my neck when I'm warm. The pony tail is just starting to reach my neck, so I reach to tighten it. A gentle pull, and my pony tail holder snaps. My hair falls in a thick clump down onto the back of my neck, with just the loop of my hat to keep it from suffocating me. This is a tragedy. Foot pain, calf pain, numb fingers - I can take all that. Hair on my neck? Impossible. But this is my Last Big Run! I turn back and find my torn pony tail holder and manage to tie it into a knot around my hair. Not as efficient as an undamaged elastic, and I have surely tied a large amount of my hair into this knot (ouch), but I can keep going. I feel like a marine showing my survival training. Pony tails are important.

Crisis averted, I keep moving. The miles pass quickly, in my head at least. My route will take me just past my friend and sometime running partner Ohia's house, and I had invited her to come run some miles with me. She said maybe. I know that probably means no, but I spend nine miles thinking about what we'll talk about, imagining the moment when I see her coming toward me, and other such schoolgirl daydreams. I text her often to keep her apprised of when I'll actually be in her area. She is nice enough to wait until I'm basically passing her house to tell me she's not coming out. It's the sign of a good running partner - even though she's not going to run with me today, she had the forethought to let me keep my distracting daydreams until the last minute.

My turnaround is a mile past her neighborhood. It's a nice, long downhill for a few miles. My other favorite running partner, my sister-in-law Cathy, had suggested making up things to look forward to on the return trip. I know I have a slight uphill, so I decide to walk for a short time and sip some water there. I do. It helps. Next I get to refuel. After that, at mile 16, I get to stop to refill my waters, apply sunscreen, and then treat myself to some music on my headphones.

But wait! What is that? On the ground at mile 12! It's a discarded pony tail holder! Sure, it may be covered in lice, but they can be my cheering crew! I do the unthinkable and reach down to pick it up. I tie it into my head. I have my real pony tail back. This feels fantastic.

I admit the last treat-stop doesn't go quite as planned. I somehow apply sunscreen to my arms as if I'm a blind elephant. When I get out my headphones, I drop the twist tie I use to keep them from knotting in my pouch. Being the hippie I am, I can't leave it behind. I stand there for what seems like a foot-lymphing eternity before I see where the twist tie has fallen. Meanwhile I am so excited to have a full store of water for the final four miles that I drink WAY too much of it. My stomach yells angrily at me when I start moving again.

The last four miles seem like the shortest run ever. My legs are tired, but after how far I have gone, this seems like nothing. I enjoy it. The sun is starting to get hot, but I don't mind. After panicking about a single twist tie, I pass an entire container of discarded Q-tips. I take it as a mystery. They are spread out too far to have simply been dumped, but not far enough to have been a slow leak or a path of breadcrumbs. And what was someone doing with an entire case of Q-tips on a running trail, anyway?

Then there's the braid. A perfectly cut braided section of hair, right next to the path. I'm sure it was from a Barbie, done by a young girl dreaming of becoming a hair stylist, but all I can imagine is a kindred spirit runner finally getting so tired of her long hair that she chopped it off right there in mid-run. That thought has certainly crossed my mind. Perhaps I should practice it on a Barbie first, though.

One last hill to climb and I'm home. I defy my sloshy stomach and drink a few last drinks of my water. My time is right on target, so I even let myself walk. I have run 19; I can walk for a bit and still earn my badge of awesomeness, yes? At the top of the short hill, I start running again. It doesn't matter how much one walks during a marathon; you ALWAYS run across that finish line. So, run I do.

My husband has texted me that he and the kids are in the back yard. I go straight there, ready to put my feet up and be pampered. The kids are there eating lunch, but the husband is MIA. Instead of propping my feet up, I have to go fetch Doritos and ketchup for my son (his favorite side dish), more water for my daughter. My son then has to poop, so I have to help him get his butt wiped. This is not the pampering I had imagined. I do manage to fix myself a real recovery drink in there as well. The husband does reappear eventually.

Twenty miles. Finished 30 seconds over my goal. 12'02" average pace.

Next time I do this, I'll have to go six more. Eep.

November 15

Rest day. The skin of my feet feels like I wore sandpaper socks yesterday, but otherwise I'm okay.

November 16

Six miles on the schedule, and I do it! My feet are still feeling abused (and I thought those socks were soft!), but the run otherwise feels fine. 11'11" average pace.

November 17

Yoga day. I put on a children's yoga video in the hopes that the kids will do that while I do my own thing in the background. It works for my daughter, but my son is soon weaseling his way onto my mat. Too add to the fun, he inexplicably takes off all his clothes and rests his naked butt on my yoga mat. Maybe I'll go to class next week.

November 18

Seven miles. I have such an urge not to do it. I did my 20 miles; I'm ready! Poor logic, I know. I run anyway. 11'33" pace.

November 19

Seven miles again? But this - this is the last seven treadmill miles I'll have to do. This mantra is less motivating than I'd hoped, but the miles happen. 11'19" average pace.

November 20

A relaxing Friday. For the first time in weeks, I resist the urge to ask my running friends to join me. I'm feeling very grumpy that I have to wake up early to run, to make sure I'm back in time to change guard so my husband can get to a meeting at church. As if on cue, my friend Ohia texts me in the evening to see if I'm running tomorrow. We make plans to meet up. Finally!

November 21

Just 12 miles today, and I'll get to run with Ohia for some of it. We plan it out so that I will meet her partway, and she will run five miles with me. She has done longer runs with me before, and we have even run a half marathon together, but she had a heart procedure just a few weeks ago and is just getting back from that.

The morning starts with a dose of irony; the kids that have been sleeping in until 7:00 wake up just past 6:00, right as I was about to head out the door. So, the one morning that I really have to get out the door on time so I'm not late for Ohia, I am running late. I push hard for my first few miles. The first mile is so fast, it's surely a 9'44". (It's not. It's 10'41".) It's so early that the sun isn't even touching the tops of the Catalina Mountains during my northbound mile. It gets brighter as I head south, and it crests the Rincon Mountains in the east as I reach Ohia.

It feels wonderful to run with her. We talk the whole way. The miles go quickly. I have missed this.

Today is the day of El Tour de Tucson, a major bike race that surrounds the city. The longest route in the race is just over 100 miles; our turn-around spot is on a section of the 100-mile route. According to the news, Greg Lemond will be riding in this race. When we get to the turn-around, we see him! Well, we see a guy on a bike; I don't actually know what Greg Lemond looks like now, so for all we know it could be him. A guy wearing a blue shirt riding a bike. He doesn't have a number, so we reason that Mr. Lemond is famous enough that he doesn't even have to wear a number, ergo Greg sighting. Right?

We turn back from the bicycles and begin our return route. Although the miles seem to go quickly, the clock also seems to be moving too fast. By the time we get back to Ohia's car, I realize I will have to take a short-cut to get back to my house in time for my husband to leave for his meeting. This will take a mile off my route. As I bid a thankful farewell to Ohia, I turn the math over in my head and realize that taking the short-cut will actually get me home in exactly 12 miles, and going back the way we came would give me 13. It takes me the entire run home to figure out how this happened. I somehow added an extra mile to the part I did with Ohia. I took her six miles instead of five. I took my post-heart-procedure friend a full mile longer than planned. Slow clap for me. Fast clap for her; she did just fine.

I get back to the house in time. 11'11" average pace. My husband dashes off to his meeting, only to find it starts half an hour later than he had thought. I could have had 30 more minutes of sleep. Grunt.

November 22

Rest day. Ohia and I hang out and eat fried chicken to celebrate our run.

November 23

Down to just six miles on the treadmill. It seems like so much less than seven. 11'24" pace.

November 24

Rest/yoga day. I do neither.

November 25

Last six miles on the treadmill. My husband has the day off from work, so he comes to the YMCA with us. He swims and lifts weights while I run. It's weird to have him here.

10'55" per mile.

November 26

Serendipity prevails on my training plan. This is the first (and only) day with a three-mile run. It is also the day of a 5k I like to do. It is a cross-country 5k, complete with hay bales to jump over and water (mud) features to jump across, and hundreds of runners dressed up as turkeys, pilgrims, and even a few tigers (though I'm not sure why) to celebrate the other event today: Thanksgiving. The route takes us past some man-made ponds that wintering waterfowl have come to love. I see a hundred coots, wigeons, ring-necked ducks, and even a neotropic cormorant. It is also right next to the local zoo, so as I am looking at the ducks I am being serenaded by the whoot-whoot wails of the Lars gibbons in the zoo. A strange, fun way to start the day.

The route itself is surprisingly difficult. One never notices the steep little hills in the park until one must run up them. I have great fun jumping across the hay bales. They are a warm-up for the water pits. There are two water pits to jump across, and two loops in the route. As I dash down the hill toward the water pits on the first loop, I am all ready to leap across them as I had in previous years, when suddenly everyone in front of me comes to a complete stop at them. Are they wider than last year? Why have we stopped? The spectators tell them to just run through them, and some of the runners do. Now it's my turn. I have completely lost all the momentum I had built up, but I really didn't want to splash THROUGH the mud, especially with another mile and a half to run. That pleasure is reserved for a different kind of race (and a different kind of runner). So, from a complete stop, I jump. I must be as graceful as a chicken flying over a manure heap. One of the spectators yells, "Nice jump!" I'm pretty sure the comment is meant ironically, and probably with a helping of disappointment as my foot lands dryly on the other side of the pit. I pick up a quick jog and leap across the second one.

I run around the second loop feeling a bit self-conscious that I had jumped rather than splashed, and wondering why no one else was jumping across them this year. When I come around to the mud pits this time, I see that I have no choice. So many people have splashed through them that the far sides are nothing but slippery mud. If I attempt to jump, my foot will slide out from under me and I'll end up butt-first in the water. This sounds like less fun than just having wet feet for the last tenth of a mile.

So, in I go. The water is COLD, but it feels surprisingly good. I splash my left foot into the first pit, then my right foot goes in to the second. I smile as I make the last dash to the finish line. I finish in just over 32 minutes. That's just a little faster than my time for this race last year. I am also just a little wetter (okay, a LOT wetter) than last year.

I always pack a pair of flip flops to change into when I'm finished a race. Always. Except for today, of course. I drive home with sopping wet shoes. It was worth it.

November 27

Rest day.

November 28

Also a rest day. All the long runs I've been doing on Saturdays were based on a training plan that assumed a Saturday race. My race is actually on a Sunday. Next Sunday, to be exact.

Sorry, I fainted. Anyway, my race is next Sunday, so I figure I will do the last week of the training plan exactly as called for on the schedule. My last long run is a week from my race, so that should happen tomorrow.

November 29

My plan of getting up to do my last long run (just eight miles) stops as soon as I see that it's about 28 degrees outside. No reason to crawl out of my nice warm bed to run in the semi-dark and then rush to get ready for church.

It seems sudden that I can now go for a run in the daylight in Tucson without combusting, but here we are. The magic of November. We go to church, come home, and THEN I run. It is 10:30 in the morning when I head out the door. Just a month ago that could have spelled certain death. Instead, it's rather pleasant. There are dozens of other runners and cyclists on the path. While my body is wholly against running right in the middle of the mid-morning slump, I still enjoy the run. I even picture the finish line a few times. I'll finish my run today around noon; that's also about when I expect to cross the finish line next week.

I pay attention to the little details. My legs are hot in my long pants right now; I decide shorts are the way to go next week. The sun is so bright that it seems to erase all the colors of the desert; I must NOT forget my sunglasses next week. I stop for a sip of water after seven miles, and it manages to rehydrate a hideous layer of slime on my tongue; I must drink water more frequently next week, whether I am thirsty or not. (Also, seriously eew!)

11'30" per mile. If I do that next week, I will not make my 5-hour dream time.

November 30

Rest day. I look to the Internet for suggestions on what to eat the week before a marathon. I am frightened by the amount of carbs I am supposed to eat. Not that I'm against carbs in general; it's just SO much! I dutifully dump a pile of pretzels next to my yogurt for lunch, and I turn the last leftover mashed potatoes from Thanksgiving into potato bread to go aside tonight's chili.

December 1

I only have to run four miles today. How decadent!
11'06" average pace. I have a bagel with lunch.

December 2

Rest day. Burritos and crackers and cereal, oh my!

December 3

Four miles, miles 2-3 at marathon pace.

December 4

Rest again. They could just as easily call these
"overthinking days" instead of rest days.

December 5

Twenty-five minutes of running. Since it's a Saturday
and the drive to packet pick-up will take us past one of my
favorite restaurants, we all pile into the car to make a day of
it. I order my favorite pasta, only to find they have taken it off
the menu. The server talks me into an alternative pasta
dish, to which I acquiesce. Instead of being light and
tomato-y like my old favorite, this one has an alfredo sauce
that sits in my stomach like a greasy brick. Since the
restaurant is also a fantastic brewery, we bring along a
growler to fill with some of my favorite celebratory
beverages. We are told, however, that by Arizona law, I am
not allowed to take any of their good brews home in the
growler. We leave with something mediocre, and I try not to

allow my mind to consider this double-downfall of plans to be a bad omen.

The packet pick-up is quick and efficient. I proudly wear my Cape May Point 5-mile t-shirt, knowing this race was way more meaningful than all the marathon and ultramarathon (What on earth is that? 50k? 50 miles?! I'm NEVER doing something like that!) t-shirts I see in the room. I feel vaguely lightheaded when I stand at the full-marathon check-in. This feeling is replaced with confidence as I look at the route map posted on the wall. I know where I'm going. I know what I'm doing. I'm ready for this.

Except, of course, I still have a dozen things to do. As this is a Sunday race, I will be missing church. I still bake cookies, as I do most weeks, with the plan to send them in with my husband. I have time for two loads of laundry. I dutifully shower and shave my legs as closely as possible to avoid chafing. The layer of skin I take off on my inner thighs will surely help, yes?

My clothes are laid out. My water bottles (the hippie in me cannot handle 26.2 miles of disposable paper cups) are filled and in the fridge. My alarm is set for a disturbingly early hour.

I'm ready as I'll ever be.

December 6

Race Day.

After a fitful night of sleep filled with every race dream imaginable (going off-course, forgetting shoes, forgetting clothes at all, forgetting I even have a marathon and going to IHOP instead…), I wake up five minutes before my 3:15 alarm. I force down a bagel with peanut butter, drink my coffee with all its poopful magic, and stare at the banana I had laid out. Between nerves and the early morning, my stomach is unenthusiastic about breakfast; I stash the banana in my drop bag for later.

A goodbye grunt from my still-sleeping husband, and I'm out the door. It is about a 45 minute drive to the full marathon parking area. I'm nervous that I won't find it, but as I get closer, the road goes from empty to being crowded with cars with their "26.2" stickers. My husband has made fun of my 13.1 sticker, but I find such comfort in these cars telling me I'm in the right place, I vow to put a 26.2 on my car as soon as I get home. I follow the stickers to a well-lit parking lot and two or three buses. I board the bus. It fills quickly, and we're off.

I try to sit back and enjoy the now-familiar race-bus smell of menthol and methane. Sore muscles and nervous intestines, and the need to rattle off each race one has ever done. The bus drives for what seems like hours. Eventually we start pulling into the hills where the race begins. I can see the outlines of small trees in the moonlight; we have gained quite a bit in elevation. It will be fun to run down this.

And we park. I stay on the bus for a bit to keep warm. I take out my banana and give it a long, hard stare, then place it back into my bag. The bag that doesn't have my water bottles in it, as they are still at home in the fridge. Bad hippie.

After a while I get off the bus to get in line for the bathroom. This is the most stressful part of the race. Everyone is eager to poop the best poop they can. The lines are long. Some folks are well-hydrated enough that the lines are TOO long. Lots of shadows are squatting in the desert on either side of the road. A man cuts into the line. Tempers flare, but a woman speaks to him with the poise and patient logic of a kindergarten teacher explaining why a child cannot act the way he has. Tail between his legs, the man moves to the back of a (different) line.

As I wait in line, announcements are being made. Announcements that the group who arrived on a certain bus should get onto the front bus immediately. It seems one of the bus drivers for the half marathon has accidentally driven his group up to the full marathon start. I cannot imagine the stress these folks are feeling. After a while these announcements are replaced by requests for the driver of that front bus to get back on the bus to drive them to the correct place. These announcements are made repeatedly and with ever-increasing desperation. The drama is palpable.

Business completed, I move to a table to start pinning my bib on. I'm irritated by the feel of it crinkling when I sit, so I generally wait until the last minute to put it on. I lay out my safety pins and attempt to get it as straight as possible. I get two of them on when volunteers come over and say they have to move the table right away. Apparently the rogue bus driver has been located, but the table must be moved for the bus to get by. I grab my things off the table and get out of the way hastily. The bus makes its exit, and I realize I have lost a safety pin.

The sky starts to glow in the east, and the outlines of giant boulders start to form. We are at about 5,000' above sea level, tucked against the Santa Catalina Mountains. At this level there are tiny live-oak trees that also start to sneak out of the shadows of night. The start is delayed slightly so that the busload of half marathoners can make it to their start line.

I dance in place to keep from getting too cold. It's a small group. No need for corrals here. I look for the 4:55 pacer, but he or she is not here. I have a choice between 4:40 (unlikely) and 5:30 (please no!). I plant myself between the two. I see a man dressed as Superman. Several people wearing tutus. Most bizarre of all, a guy wearing a jacket that says "American River 50 Mile". (FIFTY miles? NEVER doing that. Nice jacket, though.)

It's been hurry-up-and-wait the whole morning. The whole five months, really. But here we are. National Anthem plays. Starting pistol starts. And we're off! I am doing it - I am running a marathon!

I am running a marathon FAST. The first part is wonderfully downhill. I rock it. I slow only to watch a handful of birds (Bridled Titmice - not something I'll get to see once we drop elevation), then tear it up down the road some more. 5:30 is a distant memory. 4:40 is visible in front of me on the straighter sections of roads. I am running fast. I am not running smart.

We pass through the town of Oracle. This place is awesome. I see several of my dream homes, tucked away in the wilderness on the quiet side of the mountains. A man is waving a huge American flag at us all. There is a gorgeous stone building with a National Register of Historic Places plaque out front; I haven't seen one of those since I was in New Jersey! We pass a grouping of several tiny A-frames, so very out of place in Arizona, that is apparently both a motel as well as the local locksmith. Down the hill a bit more is a cafe with outdoor seating, and a waitress bringing out a platter of sizzling bacon to smarter-than-us breakfast patrons.

10'45" first mile. 10'53". 10'46". I am on fire, I stupidly think.

The course starts to flatten out a bit. We start seeing signs of more generalized civilization. We pass a Dollar General and a Circle K convenience store, both of which have an amusing number of people wearing marathon bibs coming in and out of them. 11'27". 10'57". I see my friend Ohia at the first baton-exchange point for the marathon relay; she will be running the last part but must go with her entire team to each exchange point. She cheers me on. I hope I'm not already finished by the time her team reaches the last leg.10'45". 10'38". I am unstoppable.

The course turns out onto State Route 77. Up here it's just a two-lane road with a sweeping view of desert to the right and the mountains to the left. 11'15". It's still downhill, but not as much as before. 11'07". I get a text from Cathy cheering me on. I can't believe how good I feel. I shouldn't believe how good I feel.

The sun is now all the way up, and it's starting to get a bit warm. I wish I had not forgotten my water bottles. 11'14". The route turns up toward Biosphere II. I know this area well; it's the start of the half marathon. I'm just about halfway. We will go up this road for a bit, then turn around and head back. The road is a roller coaster. The downs feel good, but the ups are starting to feel a bit excruciating. 11'57". Ever-giving, ever-supporting Cathy is planning on meeting me on her bike at the end of the road on my way back out. 12'40". I see her. I love her.

Cathy rides with me down the hill. The people around me mention how lucky I am to have her. I am lucky! She takes my arm warmers (was I seriously freezing cold just a couple of hours ago?) and puts them in her bag. She hands me an anti-chafe stick (another thing I forgot this morning) to rub on my already-bleeding over-shaved thigh. There is so much desert dust on my legs by now, this does nothing but make her chafe stick dirty. Sorry, Cathy. 11'53". Halfway. She hands me a full bottle of water, and I drink it all gladly. 12'21".

The course is now back out on Route 77. Oracle Road. It's barely downhill now, and there is even a pancake-flat mile coming. I really don't want to say this word, even in my own head, but it's true - I'm…. tired. I start doing the bargain-walk. I'll walk, I tell my legs, but only up to the next traffic cone. 12'22". I'll walk, but only so I can adjust my pack. 13'02. We get to the point where Cathy has parked her car, and she bids me farewell. I am so thankful to have had her.

I have no idea how I'll do the rest of this without her.

I'm by myself now. Literally. I don't see anyone in front of me, and I can barely see one person behind me. 12'09". I know I'm not lost; I've been on this section before, and it's all just a single road.

My legs might hate me.

14'01". I'm at mile 18. Everyone says this is the hardest mile of the marathon. You've been running a long time, so you're tired, but you're not exactly close to the finish either. I'm fighting to make myself run. I take more short walk breaks. 15'11". 15'14".

I'm at the back of the pack. I can barely see people behind me. But I'm at mile 20. I've heard it said that a marathon is a 20-mile run followed by a 10k race. I have no idea how anyone would feel like racing at this point. I'm barely running. I slow down to put in my headphones. While I don't usually listen to headphones on non-treadmill runs, I had promised myself that I could listen to headphones from mile 20-25, just to get me through those last few miles. As I slow down and dig around in my wastepack to find my headphones, a course volunteer on a bicycle rolls over to ask if I'm okay. I tell him I'm great; I finally earned my music. The care in his voice, however, tells me how far back I am and how tired I must look.

The music works for a bit. I listen to the same playlist I had listened to on my runs in New Jersey. For a few moments I am transported back to the cool shadows of trees, but the harsh reality of the unseasonably hot desert sun (it's now getting up past 80) cuts through that reverie quickly. I keep pushing. 13'40". 13'45. Not terrible. Not good, either.

I do have a few other exhausted people near me now. The course turns off of the main road to go through some lovely neighborhoods, and up that stupid hill on which I have no plans whatsoever of running. I make it to the top. It's not even a large hill; just a minute of walking and I'm there. It feels like climbing the lighthouse at this point. We cross a street, and policemen are there to keep us safe. They have been there for us this entire time, and I have been calling out "thank you" to them as I passed. This time, however, another exhausted soul near me calls out, "Thank you! We wouldn't be able to look for traffic at this point!" And I realize he's right. I am so exhausted, I don't think I could actually turn my head left or right to see if any cars were coming, and I'm not sure my mind would register it even if I saw one.

My body hurts. I have given birth twice. That was fun. It was a fun pain. This is not a fun pain. I feel like everything in my body is being crushed. Once in high school a genius friend of mine took a pair of super-strong magnets and made a nose-ring out of them. In an instant he was shrieking in pain trying to get them out. I feel like those magnets are all over my body, haphazardly squishing parts of me. Why do I feel like this? I know I trained well. I ran all the running I needed to run to run this. Did I not do enough yoga? I settle on that fault. It's an easy fault on which to settle, given that I am growing a horn out of the back of my neck. At least, I feel like I must be. I'm too tired to reach up and feel for it. It's not a beautiful unicorn horn, either. An ugly, calciferous growth, straight out the base of the back of my neck. It's so stiff, I can feel it in my neck, shoulders, and upper back.

I am down to a walk. Walking is not even easier than running. Walking is just as hard. 16'18". Time to take out my headphones for the last mile. At this point I forget why I had decided to do that. Was it so I could hear the finish line as I got closer? Or so I looked better in my finish line photos? I have no idea. I just remember I wanted to take them out, so I take them out.

For the last few miles, people have been passing me. I can hear them catching easily up to me. The sound pains me until the last minute when I see that their bibs are a different color - they are running the last leg of the relay. They only have a few miles to run. Their legs are fresh. Still, I am coming to hate the sound of their easy pace. (Another tired runner later remarks that the race directors were smart to color-code the bib, or all us back-of-the-packers would surely have intentionally tripped those happy fresh faces.) To add to this irritation, I start to see blue bibs like mine walking smugly in the other direction. Folks who have finished. That'll be me soon, right? I try to excite myself. But then I see it.

The medal.

It's hideous.

It's a saguaro. The symbol of my exile. (Okay, Tucson isn't so bad, but I admit I'm definitely not loving it so much right now.) Not only that, it's RED (my second-least favorite color) with orangey-red triangles (my least favorite color) on it. It is the most ugly, evil thing I have ever seen. My body feels like this so I can have THAT piece of hatred.

I start to cry.

But, nowhere to go but forward. So I press on. I am surprised to realize that I am about to overtake someone. There is someone walking toward the finish line, slowly but methodically. She is large. Very large. It's a different enough scene that I wonder for a moment if it's a spectator who has wandered out onto the course thinking the race is all done. As I pass, though, I manage to turn around and see a different color bib - this person is just finishing the half marathon! The way she moves, step by determined step, despite her size, is absolutely inspirational. A wave of joy washes away the negative feelings I had just felt. This full marathon I'm doing is nothing compared to the feat this lady is about to accomplish. I say, "Good job!" as I pass her. She smiles.

Last full mile. 16'24". I have two corners to turn. The first brings me onto the road on which the finish area is located, and the second leads the last few yards to the finish line. It's close. I can hear it. (Good thing I took my headphones off.)

I stopped looking at my phone ages ago to see how much I had slowed down. I turn the last corner and finally see the race clock. It's reading 5:40. My dream goal was under 5. My realistic goal was 5:15. My desperate goal was less than 5:24. I'm well past all of that.

I'm just a few yards from the finish, and I want to stop. I want a DNF. I don't want this time. I want to quit.

My husband and kids are there. I feel bad quitting right in front of them. But then I see her - Ohia! Ohia must have finished AGES ago. She's on a team of folks from her job, none of whom know me, but all of whom have been standing there with her waiting for me to finish.

That's when I know I HAVE to finish.

I wave to my unfortunate fans and jog on to the finish line.

A friend had excitedly told me that crossing the finish line at my first marathon would be one of the best feelings in my life. This is quite the opposite. I cross the finish with feelings of self-loathing, misery, and embarrassment. A good-looking fireman is there to put my medal on me. I do not want him to. I hate the medal, and I don't deserve it. I reach up and take it from him and clutch it in my hand, figuring that would be easier than trying to explain to him why I don't want it. I try desperately to smile at him, and to the person who is there to take finish-line photos.

I'm done. At least I can stop running. I know I should eat, so I make my way over to the food tent. It was the birthday of the organizer's wife, or some similar person, so there are cupcakes. They are beautiful, and I have absolutely no interest in eating them. I take a little cup full of thin wheat crackers and go out to meet my husband and kids. My son eats most of my crackers, which is fine with me as it takes me five minutes to force myself to eat a single one. I never realized how much chewing is involved in eating a cracker.

Rather than take the bus back to the parking area, I ride the spectator bus back to my husband's truck. The bus ride is my son's favorite part. In the truck, my husband drives me to the parking lot where I left my car. I think. We come from the other direction, and we turn into the wrong parking lot. There are a half dozen marathoners wandering around the lot, but I don't see my car. We pull out and go to the next lot down. Again, several marathoners wandering around, but no car. We finally find my car in the third lot. I bid farewell to my kids, slide out of the truck, and hobble over to my car. More marathoners are wandering around. I hear them complaining that the buses had actually picked up people from several different but nearly identical parking lots in the morning, and no one realized it; now no one knew where their cars are. I'm thankful my husband was able to drive me around and I did not have to walk.

I mix a quick protein shake to drink on the way home. The feel of my bare legs on my fake leather seats is horrible. It will take me at least 45 minutes to get home, so I take off my shirt and slide it under my legs. Getting pulled over for driving shirtless will be nowhere near as humiliating as the marathon I just ran.

Home, showered, I sit back and think about the day. I have never hated anything as much as I hated running through the finish line. Never. So why do people do this multiple times? I must have done it wrong. If I did it wrong, I must try it again. Yes, this thing that I just detested with every inch of my soul, I must do again. That very night, thanks in part to my inability to read at this level of exhaustion (I have a coupon code that expires in ten days, but I read that as "today" - act now!), I sign up for the Phoenix Marathon in two months. That will hold me over for the short term. There is no way I could wait for an entire year to figure this out; I know I need to do Phoenix. That is a different course, however, in a different place. I need to try this one again and see what I did wrong here. So, as soon as registration opens, I sign up for next year.

Less than 72 hours after this loathsome event, I am signed up for two more.

Epilogue

The Phoenix Marathon was different. Cathy wanted to run it with me, so she did. We stayed in a hotel, so I avoided the pitfalls of attempting to finish housework instead of relaxing. My only time goal this time was to finish in six hours - and that simply because the website said they would be handing out medals up until that time. The website was polite enough to post a picture of the medal, so I knew it was not one that would make me suddenly start sobbing.

After her injury, Cathy had a genius scheme of walking every sixth mile. That would still put us well within the six hour cutoff, so I agreed happily. We started out just before dawn in the gorgeous Usery Pass area. It was a chilly February morning when we started, but it soon heated up to record-high heat. The walking breaks were welcome, as were the extra baggies of ice volunteers were handing out. We kept up a steady pace for the first half, barring some newlywed delays; Cathy's husband met us several times for water, blister care, wardrobe adjustments, and the requisite newlywed kissing time. All told, according to my running app, we spent fifteen minutes standing still. That made the day fifteen minutes hotter, though. At mile 17, when a complete stranger was on the side of the road offering cold Cokes and Twinkies, I happily took the Coke. (Coke is now one of my staple running fuels.) We slowed quite a bit toward the end because Cathy had a very nasty blister (and then lost that blister, to the chorus of some words I didn't know were in her vocabulary). They were starting to reopen the roads. I was nervous I would miss my time goal, but then the finish line was in sight. I sprinted joyfully toward it. My kids, now sporting cowbells, were there cheering me on. My husband, now sporting the face of a guy whose kids now have cowbells, was watching with a smile only wives and the makers of Excedrin could love. Music was playing. My legs were alive. Just one more dash, and done! I had finished my second marathon - and beat my time goal by 32 seconds! One volunteer spread two cold, wet washcloths on my shoulders while another placed the medal over my head. I took it all like Miss America receiving her crown and flowers. This was the best feeling on Earth. THIS was why people run marathons.

And the best part? I wasn't even tired! Taking it slowly, taking breaks, drinking that magical soda… I could go on! I could keep running! I could - gasp - do a 50k…